Ophthalmology

50p

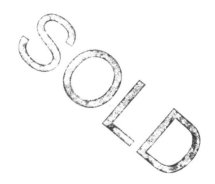

Ophthalmology

BRUCE JAMES

MA, DM, FRCS(Ed), FRCOphth
Consultant Ophthalmologist
Department of Ophthalmology
Stoke Mandeville Hospital
Buckinghamshire

CHRIS CHEW

FRCS (Glasg), FRCOphth
Consultant Ophthalmologist
Wolverhampton and Midland Counties Eye Infirmary
Wolverhampton

ANTHONY BRON

BSc FRCS, FRCOphth
Professor of Ophthalmology
Nuffield Laboratory of Ophthalmology
Oxford

Eighth Edition

b

**Blackwell
Science**

© 1960, 1965, 1968, 1971, 1974, 1980,
1986, 1997 by
Blackwell Science Ltd
Editorial Offices:
Osney Mead, Oxford OX2 0EL
25 John Street, London WC1N 2BL
23 Ainslie Place, Edinburgh EH3 6AJ
350 Main Street, Malden
   MA 02148 5018, USA
54 University Street, Carlton
   Victoria 3053, Australia
10, rue Casimir Delavigne
   75006 Paris, France

Other Editorial Offices:
Blackwell Wissenschafts-Verlag GmbH
Kurfürstendamm 57
10707 Berlin, Germany

Blackwell Science KK
MG Kodenmacho Building
7-10 Kodenmacho Nihombashi
Chuo-ku, Tokyo 104, Japan

The right of the Author to be
identified as the Author of this Work
has been asserted in accordance
with the Copyright, Designs and
Patents Act 1988.

First published 1960
Reprinted 1961, 1963
Second edition 1965
Third edition 1968
Fourth edition 1971
Fifth edition 1974
Reprinted 1976
Spanish edition 1978
Sixth edition 1980
Seventh edition 1986
Eighth edition 1997
Reprinted 1998

Set by Excel Typesetters Co., Hong Kong
Printed and bound in Italy
by Vincenzo Bona srl, Turin

The Blackwell Science logo is a
trade mark of Blackwell Science Ltd,
registered at the United Kingdom
Trade Marks Registry

DISTRIBUTORS

Marston Book Services Ltd
PO Box 269
Abingdon, Oxon OX14 4YN
(Orders: Tel: 01235 465500
          Fax: 01235 465555)
USA
Blackwell Science, Inc.
Commerce Place
350 Main Street
Malden, MA 02148 5018
(Orders: Tel: 800 759 6102
               781 388 8250
          Fax: 781 388 8255)
Canada
Login Brothers Book Company
324 Saulteaux Crescent
Winnipeg, Manitoba R3J 3T2
(Orders: Tel: 204 224-4068)
Australia
Blackwell Science Pty Ltd
54 University Street
Carlton, Victoria 3053
(Orders: Tel: 3 9347 0300
          Fax: 3 9347 5001)

A catalogue record for this title
is available from the British Library

ISBN 0-86542-723-2 (BSL)
     0-632-04154-4 (IE)

Library of Congress
Cataloguing-in-publication Data

James, Bruce, 1957-
   Lecture notes on ophthalmology. — 8th ed. /
Bruce James, Chris Chew, Anthony Bron.
          p.   cm. — (Lecture notes series)
   Rev. ed. of: Lecture notes on ophthalology /
Patrick D. Trevor-Roper. 7th ed. 1986.
   Includes bibliographical references
and index
   ISBN 0-86542-723-2
   I. Ophthalmology — Outlines, syllabi, etc.
I. Chew, Chris.   II. Bron, Anthony J.
III. Trevor-Roper, Patrick Dacre, 1916–
Lecture notes on ophthalmology.   IV. Title.
   [DNLM: I. Eye Diseases.
WW 140 J27L   1996]
RE50.T73   1996
617.7 — dc20
DNLM/DLC
for Library of Congress   96-20972
                                                CIP

For further information on Blackwell Science,
visit our website: www.blackwell-science.com

Contents

Preface to eighth edition

Much has changed in ophthalmology since the first edition of this book in 1960, written by the distinguished ophthalmologist Patrick Trevor-Roper. We are honoured to follow in his footsteps. Ophthalmology still remains something of a medical 'Cinderella' afforded little time in a busy medical student's timetable. Yet eye disease accounts for a substantial number of consultations in general practice and cataract surgery is recognized as one of the most successful operations in the surgical armamentarium. Furthermore, many systemic medical diseases have ocular manifestations. As Patrick Trevor-Roper wrote in his introduction:

> To the ancients, the eye was the gateway for the soul, and to the physician of today that modest organ indeed serves as a window through which the evidence can be seen of half the maladies to which man is heir.

The medical curriculum is nonetheless vast and time not unlimited for the busy medical student. Each specialty must try to distil the essence of the subject, which is the principal aim of the lecture notes series.

In this edition of lecture notes we have been fortunate in the development of printing techniques which have greatly reduced the costs of reproducing illustrations and drawings. Ophthalmology remains a subject where diagnosis depends on appearance rather than investigation, thus the ability to include numerous illustrations is of enormous benefit. We have changed the layout of the book to consider disease as it affects the different tissues of the eye rather than the major symptoms of ocular disease. Appendices have been included, however, which detail the differential diagnosis of these major symptoms. We hope that these lecture notes will help to unravel some of the mystery that still seems to surround ophthalmology and make the short time spent in the eye department an enjoyable and useful one.

Bruce James
Chris Chew
Anthony Bron

Preface to first edition

This little guide does not presume to tell the medical student all that he needs to know about ophthalmology, for there are many larger books that do. But the medical curriculum becomes yearly more congested, while ophthalmology, still the 'Cinderella' of medicine, is generally left until the last, and only too readily goes by default. So it is to these harrassed final-year students that the book is principally offered, in the sincere hope that they will find it useful; for nearly all eye diseases are recognized quite simply by their appearance, and a guide to ophthalmology need be little more than a gallery of pictures, linked by lecture notes.

My second excuse for publishing these lecture notes is a desire I have always had to escape from the traditional textbook presentation of ophthalmology as a string of small isolated diseases, with long unfamiliar names, and a host of eponyms. To the nineteenth-century empiricist, it seemed proper to classify a long succession of ocular structures, all of which emerged as isolated brackets for yet another sub-catalogue of small and equally isolated diseases. Surely it is time now to try and harness these miscellaneous ailments, not in terms of their diverse morphology, but in simpler clinical patterns; not as the microscopist lists them, but in the different ways that eye diseases present. For this, after all, is how the student will soon be meeting them.

I am well aware of the many inadequacies and omissions in this form of presentation, but if the belaboured student finds these lecture notes at least more readable, and therefore more memorable, than the prolix and time-honoured pattern, perhaps I will be justified.

Patrick Trevor-Roper

Acknowledgements

The hunt for illustrations can be arduous, the authors are thus particularly grateful to: Richard Bates, Larry Benjamin, Hung Cheng, John Elston, Peggy Frith, James Hsuan, Ramona Khooshabah, Brendan McDonald, Tom Meagher and John Salmon for allowing us to use clinical pictures in this book. We also thank Paul Parker for his technical skill in taking many of these clinical pictures.

Numerous colleagues have provided valuable advice in their specialist areas. We are particularly grateful to our medical student reviewers Russell Young and Parminder Ghura who made numerous thoughtful and valuable comments.

Andrew Robinson has proved to be an editor of remarkable patience in awaiting the arrival of the manuscript and the illustrator and production staff at Blackwell Science have been extremely efficient in putting the book together.

Bruce James
Chris Chew
Anthony Bron

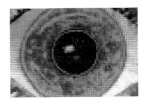

Anatomy

INTRODUCTION

A knowledge of ocular anatomy and function is important to the understanding of eye diseases. A brief outline is given below.

GROSS ANATOMY (Fig. 1.1)

The eye comprises:

• A tough outer coat which is transparent anteriorly (the *cornea*) and opaque posteriorly (the *sclera*). The junction between the two is called the *limbus*. The extraocular muscles attach to the sclera while the optic nerve leaves the sclera posteriorly through the *cribriform plate*.

• A rich vascular coat (the *choroid*) lines the posterior segment of the eye and nourishes the retina at its inner surface.

• The *ciliary body* lies anteriorly. It contains the smooth *ciliary muscle* whose contraction alters lens shape and enables the focus of the eye to be changed. The ciliary epithelium secretes *aqueous humour* and maintains the ocular pressure. The ciliary body provides attachment for the *iris*.

• The *lens* lies behind the iris and is supported by fine fibrils (the *zonule*) running between the lens and the ciliary body.

• The angle formed by the iris and cornea (the *iridocorneal angle*) is lined by a meshwork of cells and collagen beams (the *trabecular meshwork*). In the sclera outside this, *Schlemm's canal* conducts the aqueous humour from the anterior chamber into the venous system permitting aqueous drainage. This region is termed the *drainage angle*.

Between the cornea anteriorly and the lens and iris posteriorly lies the *anterior chamber*. Between the iris, the lens and the ciliary body lies the *posterior chamber* (which is distinct from the *vitreous body*). Both these chambers are filled with aqueous humour. Between the lens and the retina lies the vitreous body.

Anteriorly, the *conjunctiva* is reflected from the sclera onto the underside of the upper and lower eyelids. A connective tissue layer (*Tenon's capsule*) separates the conjunctiva from the sclera and is prolonged backwards as a sheaf around the rectus muscles.

ANATOMY OF THE EYE

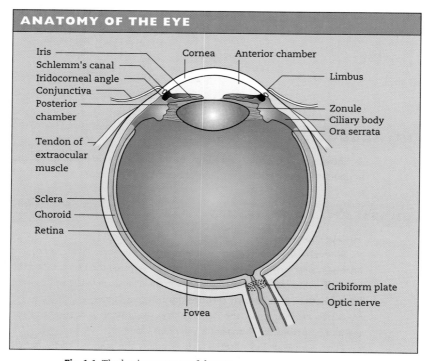

Fig. 1.1 The basic anatomy of the eye.

ORBIT (Fig. 1.2)

The eye lies within a bony orbit whose structure is shown opposite. The orbit has the shape of a four-sided pyramid. At its posterior apex is the *optic canal* which transmits the optic nerve to the brain. The *superior and inferior orbital fissures* allow the passage of blood vessels and cranial nerves to the orbit. On the anterior medial wall lies a fossa for the *lacrimal sac*. The *lacrimal gland* lies anteriorly in the superolateral aspect of the orbit.

ANATOMY OF THE ORBIT

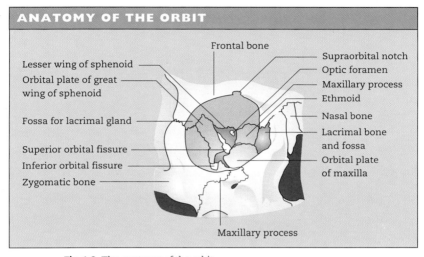

Frontal bone
Supraorbital notch
Optic foramen
Maxillary process
Ethmoid
Nasal bone
Lacrimal bone and fossa
Orbital plate of maxilla

Lesser wing of sphenoid
Orbital plate of great wing of sphenoid
Fossa for lacrimal gland
Superior orbital fissure
Inferior orbital fissure
Zygomatic bone

Maxillary process

Fig. 1.2 The anatomy of the orbit.

THE EYELIDS (TARSAL PLATES) (Fig. 1.3)

The eyelids:
- provide mechanical protection to the anterior globe;
- secrete the oily part of the tear film;
- spread the tear film over the conjunctiva and cornea;
- prevent drying of the eyes;
- contain the puncta through which the tears drain into the lacrimal drainage system.

  They comprise:
- A surface layer of skin.
- The *orbicularis muscle*.
- A tough collagenous layer (the *tarsal plate*).
- An epithelial lining, the conjunctiva, reflected onto the globe.

  The *levator muscle* passes forwards to the upper lid and inserts into the tarsal plate. It is innervated by the third nerve. Damage to the nerve or changes in old age result in drooping of the eyelid (*ptosis*). A flat smooth muscle arising from the deep surface of the levator inserts into the tarsal plate. It is innervated by the sympathetic nervous system. If the sympathetic supply is damaged (as in Horner's syndrome) a slight ptosis results.

The margin of the eyelid is the site of the *mucocutaneous junction*. It contains the openings of the *meibomian oil glands* which are located in the tarsal plate. These secrete the lipid component of the tear film. Medially, on the upper and lower lids, two small puncta form the initial part of the lacrimal drainage system.

ANATOMY OF THE EYELIDS

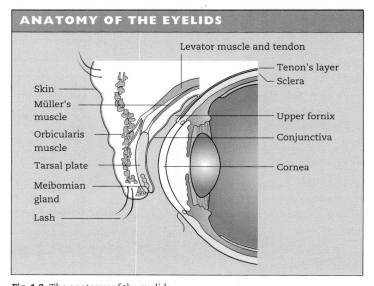

Fig. 1.3 The anatomy of the eyelids.

THE LACRIMAL DRAINAGE SYSTEM (Fig. 1.4)

Tears drain into the upper and lower *puncta* and then into the *lacrimal sac* via the upper and lower *canaliculi* which form a common canaliculus before entering the lacrimal sac. The *nasolacrimal duct* passes from the sac to the nose. Failure of the distal part of the nasolacrimal duct to fully canalize at birth is the usual cause of a watering sticky eye in a baby. Tear drainage is an active process. Each blink of the lids helps to pump tears through the system.

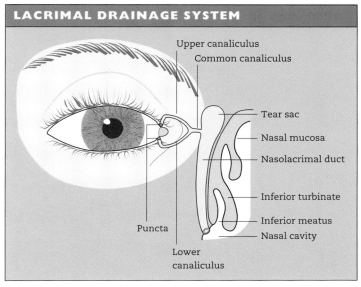

LACRIMAL DRAINAGE SYSTEM

Upper canaliculus
Common canaliculus
Tear sac
Nasal mucosa
Nasolacrimal duct
Inferior turbinate
Inferior meatus
Nasal cavity
Puncta
Lower
canaliculus

Fig. 1.4 The major components of the lacrimal drainage system.

DETAILED FUNCTIONAL ANATOMY

The tear film

The tear film (10 µm thick) covers the external ocular surface and comprises three layers:

1 a thin *mucous layer* in contact with the ocular surface and produced mainly by the conjunctival goblet cells;

2 an *aqueous layer* produced by the lacrimal gland;

3 a surface *oil layer* produced by the tarsal meibomian glands and delivered to the lid margins.

The functions of the tear film are as follows:

• it provides a smooth air/tear interface for distortion free refraction of light at the cornea;

• it provides oxygen anteriorly to the avascular cornea;

• it removes debris and foreign particles from the ocular surface through the flow of tears;

• it has antibacterial properties through the action of lysozyme, lactoferrin and the immunoglobulins, including secretory IgA.

The cornea (Fig. 1.5)

The cornea is half a millimetre thick and comprises:

- The *epithelium*, an anterior squamous layer thickened peripherally at the limbus where it is continuous with the conjunctiva. The limbus houses its germinative cells.
- An underlying *stroma* of collagen fibrils, ground substance and fibroblasts. The regular packing and small diameter of the collagen fibrils accounts for corneal transparency.
- The *endothelium*, a monolayer of non-regenerating cells which actively pumps ions and water from the stroma to control corneal hydration and clarity.

The difference between the regenerative capacity of the epithelium and endothelium is important. Damage to the epithelial layer, by an abrasion for example, is rapidly repaired. Endothelium, damaged by disease or surgery, cannot be regenerated. Loss of its barrier and pumping functions leads to overhydration, distortion of the regular packing of collagen fibres and corneal clouding.

The functions of the cornea are as follows:

- it refracts light, together with the lens it focuses light onto the retina;
- it protects the internal ocular structures.

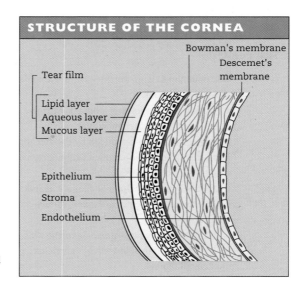

STRUCTURE OF THE CORNEA

Bowman's membrane

Descemet's membrane

Tear film

Lipid layer

Aqueous layer

Mucous layer

Epithelium

Stroma

Endothelium

Fig. 1.5 The structure of the cornea and precorneal tear film. (Schematic)

The sclera

The sclera:
- is formed from interwoven collagen fibrils of different widths and from fibroblasts and ground substance;
- is of variable thickness, 1 mm around the optic nerve head and 0.3 mm just posterior to the muscle insertions.

The choroid

The choroid (Fig. 1.6):
- is formed of arterioles, venules and a dense fenestrated capillary network;
- is loosely attached to the sclera;
- has a high blood flow;
- nourishes the deep layers of the retina and may have a role in its temperature homeostasis.

The basement membrane together with that of the retinal pigment epithelium (RPE) forms the acellular membrane, Bruch's membrane, which acts as a diffusion barrier between the choroid and the retina.

The retinal pigment epithelium

The retinal pigment epithelium (RPE):
- is formed from a single layer of cells;
- is loosely attached to the retina except at the periphery (*ora serrata*) and around the optic disc;
- forms microvilli which project between the outer segment discs of the rods and cones;

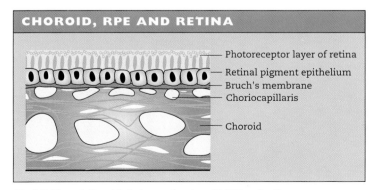

CHOROID, RPE AND RETINA

Photoreceptor layer of retina
Retinal pigment epithelium
Bruch's membrane
Choriocapillaris

Choroid

Fig. 1.6 The relationship between the choroid, RPE and retina.

- phagocytoses the redundant external segments of the rods and cones;
- facilitates the passage of nutrients and metabolites between retina and choroid;
- takes part in the regeneration of rhodopsin and cone opsin, the photoreceptor visual pigments.

The retina (Fig. 1.7)

The retina:
- Is a highly complex structure divided into ten separate layers comprising photoreceptors (*rods and cones*) and neurones, some of which (the *ganglion cells*) give rise to the optic nerve fibres.
- Is responsible for converting light into electrical signals. The initial integration of these signals is also performed by the retina.

Cones are responsible for daylight vision. Subgroups of cones are responsive to different short, medium and long wavelengths (blue, green, red). They are concentrated at the fovea which is responsible for detailed vision such as reading fine print.

Rods are responsible for night vision. They are sensitive to light and do

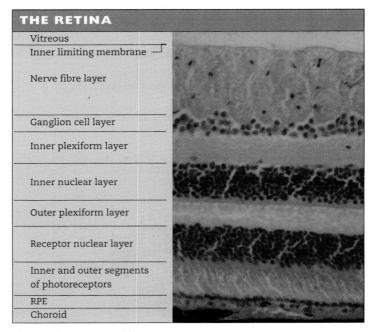

THE RETINA

Vitreous
Inner limiting membrane
Nerve fibre layer
Ganglion cell layer
Inner plexiform layer
Inner nuclear layer
Outer plexiform layer
Receptor nuclear layer
Inner and outer segments of photoreceptors
RPE
Choroid

Fig. 1.7 The structure of the retina.

not signal wavelength information (colour). They form the large majority of photoreceptors in the remaining retina.

The vitreous

The vitreous:
- Is a clear gel occupying two-thirds of the globe.
- Is 98% water. The remainder consists of hyaluronic acid and a fine collagen network. There are few cells.
- Is firmly attached anteriorly to the peripheral retina, pars plana and around the optic disc, and less firmly to the macula and retinal vessels.
- Has a nutritive and supportive role.

Detachment of the vitreous from the retina, which commonly occurs in later life, increases traction on the points of firm attachment. This may occasionally lead to a retinal break, when the vitreous pulls away a piece of the underlying retina.

The ciliary body (Fig. 1.8)

This is subdivided into three parts:
1 the *ciliary muscle*;
2 the ciliary processes (*pars plicata*);
3 the *pars plana*.

THE CILIARY MUSCLE

This:
- Comprises smooth muscle arranged in a ring overlying the ciliary processes.
- Is innervated by the parasympathetic system via the third cranial nerve.
- Is responsible for changes in lens thickness and curvature during *accommodation*. The *zonular fibres* supporting the lens are under tension during distant viewing. Contraction of the muscle relaxes them and permits the lens to increase its curvature and hence its refractive power.

THE CILIARY PROCESSES (PARS PLICATA)

There are about 70 radial *ciliary processes* arranged in a ring around the posterior chamber. They are responsible for the secretion of aqueous humour.
- Each ciliary process is formed by an epithelium two layers thick (the outer *pigmented* and inner *non-pigmented*) with a vascular stroma.
- The stromal capillaries are fenestrated, allowing plasma constituents ready access.

ANATOMY OF THE CILIARY BODY

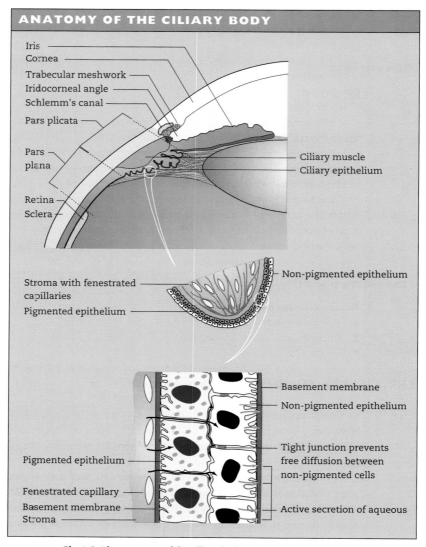

Iris
Cornea
Trabecular meshwork
Iridocorneal angle
Schlemm's canal
Pars plicata
Pars plana
Retina
Sclera

Ciliary muscle
Ciliary epithelium

Stroma with fenestrated capillaries
Pigmented epithelium
Non-pigmented epithelium

Basement membrane
Non-pigmented epithelium
Tight junction prevents free diffusion between non-pigmented cells
Pigmented epithelium
Active secretion of aqueous
Fenestrated capillary
Basement membrane
Stroma

Fig. 1.8 The anatomy of the ciliary body.

- The *tight junctions* between the non-pigmented epithelial cells provide a barrier to free diffusion into the posterior chamber. This is essential for the production of aqueous.
- The epithelial cells show marked infolding, which significantly increases their surface area for fluid and solute transport.

THE PARS PLANA

- This comprises a relatively avascular stroma covered by an epithelial layer two cells thick.
- It is safe to make surgical incisions through the scleral wall here to gain access to the vitreous cavity.

The iris

The iris:

- is attached peripherally to the anterior part of the ciliary body;
- forms the *pupil* at its centre, the aperture of which can be varied by the *sphincter* and *dilator* muscles to control the amount of light entering the eye;
- has an anterior border layer of fibroblasts and collagen and a cellular stroma in which the sphincter muscle is embedded at the pupil margin.

The smooth dilator muscle extends from the iris periphery towards the pupil. It is innervated by the sympathetic system.

The sphincter muscle is innervated by the parasympathetic system.

Posteriorly the iris is lined with a pigmented epithelium two layers thick.

The iridocorneal (drainage) angle

This lies between the iris, cornea and the ciliary body. It is the site of aqueous drainage from the eye via the trabecular meshwork.

THE TRABECULAR MESHWORK (Fig. 1.9)

This overlies Schlemm's canal and is composed of collagen beams covered by trabecular cells. The spaces between these beams become increasingly small as Schlemm's canal is approached. This meshwork accounts for most of the resistance to aqueous outflow. Damage here is thought to be the cause of the raised intraocular pressure in primary open angle glaucoma. Some of the spaces may be blocked and there is a reduction in the number of cells covering the trabecular beams (see Chapter 10).

Fluid passes into Schlemm's canal both through vacuoles in its endothelial lining and through intercellular spaces.

The lens (Fig. 1.10)

The lens:

- Is the second major refractive element of the eye, the cornea, with its tear film, is the first.

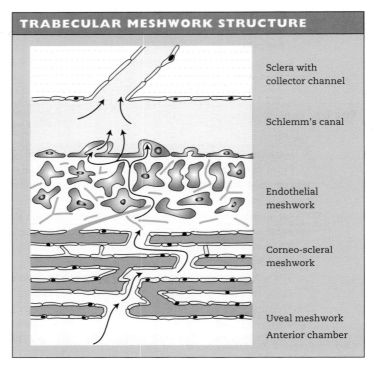

TRABECULAR MESHWORK STRUCTURE

Sclera with collector channel

Schlemm's canal

Endothelial meshwork

Corneo-scleral meshwork

Uveal meshwork
Anterior chamber

Fig. 1.9 The anatomy of the trabecular meshwork.

- Grows throughout life.
- Is supported by zonular fibres running between the lens capsule and the ciliary body.
- Comprises an outer collagenous capsule under whose anterior part lies a monolayer of epithelial cells. Towards the *equator* the epithelium gives rise to the lens fibres.

The zonular fibres transmit changes in the ciliary muscle allowing the lens to change its shape and refractive power.

The lens fibres make up the bulk of the lens. They are elongated cells arranged in layers which arch over the lens equator. Anteriorly and posteriorly they meet to form the lens *sutures*. With age the deeper *fibres* lose their nuclei and intracellular organelles.

The oldest fibres are found centrally and form the lens *nucleus*; the peripheral fibres make up the lens *cortex*.

The high refractive index of the lens arises from the high protein content of the fibres.

ANATOMY OF THE LENS

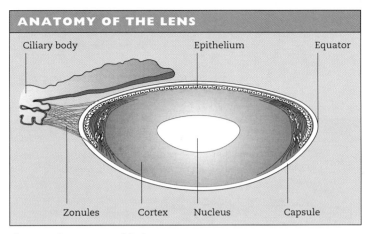

Ciliary body   Epithelium   Equator

Zonules   Cortex   Nucleus   Capsule

Fig. 1.10 The anatomy of the lens.

The optic nerve (Fig. 1.11)

- This is formed by the axons arising from the *retinal ganglion cell layer*, the innermost layer of the retina.
- Passes out of the eye through the cribriform plate of the sclera, a sieve-like structure.
- In the orbit the optic nerve is surrounded by a sheath formed by the

STRUCTURE OF THE OPTIC NERVE

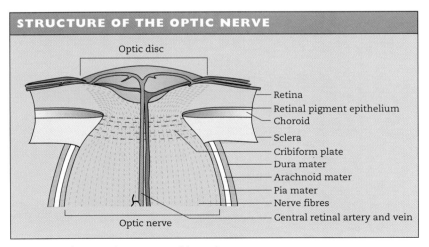

Optic disc

Retina
Retinal pigment epithelium
Choroid
Sclera
Cribiform plate
Dura mater
Arachnoid mater
Pia mater
Nerve fibres
Central retinal artery and vein

Optic nerve

Fig. 1.11 The structure of the optic nerve.

dura, arachnoid and pia mater continous with that surrounding the brain. It is bathed in cerebrospinal fluid.

The central retinal artery and vein enter the eye in the centre of the optic nerve.

The extraocular nerve fibres are myelinated; those within the eye are usually not.

THE OCULAR BLOOD SUPPLY (Fig. 1.12)

The eye receives its blood supply from the ophthalmic artery (a branch of the internal carotid artery) via the retinal artery, ciliary arteries and muscular arteries (see Fig. 1.12). The conjunctival circulation anastomoses anteriorly with branches from the external carotid artery.

The anterior optic nerve is supplied by branches from the ciliary arteries. The retina is supplied by arterioles branching from the central retinal artery. These arterioles each supply an area of retina with little overlap. Obstruction results in ischaemia of most of the area supplied by that arteriole. The fovea is so thin that it requires no supply from the retinal circulation. It is supplied indirectly, as are the outer layers of the retina, by diffusion of oxygen and metabolites across the retinal pigment epithelium from the choroid.

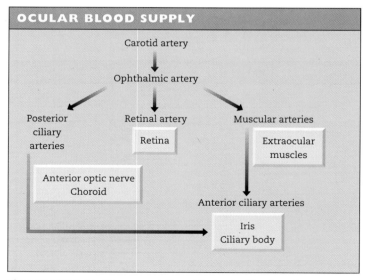

Fig. 1.12 Diagrammatic representation of the ocular blood supply.

The endothelial cells of the retinal capillaries are joined by tight junctions so that the vessels are impermeable to small molecules. This forms an inner '*blood–retinal barrier*'. The capillaries of the choroid, however, are fenestrated and leaky. The retinal pigment epithelial cells are also joined by tight junctions and present an external barrier between the leaky choroid and the retina.

It is the breakdown of these barriers that causes the retinal signs seen in many vascular diseases.

THE THIRD, FOURTH AND SIXTH CRANIAL NERVES (Fig. 1.13)

The structures supplied by each of these nerves are shown in Table 1.1.

MUSCLES AND TISSUES SUPPLIED BY THE CRANIAL NERVES

Third (Oculomotor)	Fourth (Trochlear)	Sixth (Abducens)
Medial rectus	Superior oblique	Lateral rectus
Inferior rectus		
Superior rectus (innervated by the contralateral nucleus)		
Inferior oblique		
Levator palpebrae (Both levators are innervated by a single midline nucleus.)		
Preganglionic parasympathetic fibres end in the ciliary ganglion. Here postganglionic fibres arise and pass in the short ciliary nerves to the sphincter pupillae and the ciliary muscle.		

Table 1.1 The muscles and tissues supplied by the third, fourth and sixth cranial nerves.

Central origin

The nuclei of the third (oculomotor) and fourth (trochlear) cranial nerves lie in the midbrain; the sixth nerve (abducens) nuclei lie in the pons. The diagrams show some of the important relations of these nuclei and their fascicles.

NUCLEI OF THE CRANIAL NERVES

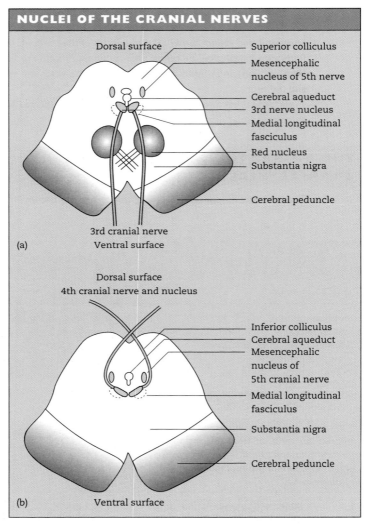

Fig. 1.13 Diagrams to show the nuclei and initial course of the (a) third and (b) fourth cranial nerves. (*Continued opposite.*)

Nuclear and fascicular palsies of these nerves are unusual. If they do occur they are associated with other neurological problems. For example if the third nerve fascicles are damaged as they pass through the red nucleus there will be a contralateral tremor as well as an ipsilateral third nerve palsy. Furthermore a nuclear third nerve lesion will result in a *con-*

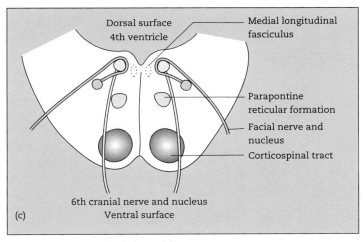

Fig. 1.13 *(Continued.)* (c) Sixth cranial nerve.

INTRACRANIAL COURSE OF THE THIRD, FOURTH AND SIXTH CRANIAL NERVES

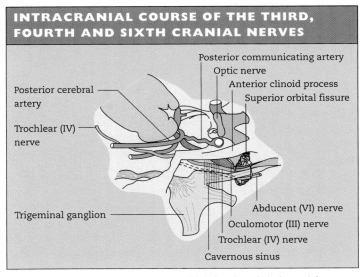

Fig. 1.14 The intracranial course of the third, fourth and sixth cranial nerves.

tralateral palsy of the superior rectus as the fibres from the subnucleus supplying this muscle cross.

Peripheral course (Fig. 1.14)

THIRD NERVE

The third nerve leaves the midbrain ventrally between the cerebral peduncles. It then passes between the *posterior cerebral* and *superior cerebellar arteries* and then lateral to the *posterior communicating artery*. Aneurysms of this artery may cause a third nerve palsy. The nerve enters the cavernous sinus in its lateral wall and enters the orbit through the superior orbital fissure.

FOURTH NERVE

The nerve decussates and leaves the *dorsal* aspect of the midbrain below the inferior colliculus. It first curves around the midbrain before passing like the third nerve between the posterior cerebral and superior cerebellar arteries to enter the lateral aspect of the cavernous sinus inferior to the third nerve. It enters the orbit via the superior orbital fissure.

SIXTH NERVE

Fibres leave from the inferior border of the pons. It has a long intracranial course passing upwards along the pons to angle anteriorly over the petrous bone and into the cavernous sinus where it lies infero-medial to the fourth nerve in proximity to the internal carotid artery. It enters the orbit through the superior orbital fissure. This long course is important because the nerve can be involved in numerous intracranial pathologies including base of skull fractures, invasion by nasopharyngeal tumours, and raised intracranial pressure.

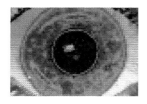

History and examination

INTRODUCTION

Ophthalmic diagnosis is heavily dependent on a good history and a thorough examination. The majority of ophthalmic diagnoses do not require additional tests.

HISTORY

A good history must include details of:
- Ocular symptoms, time of onset, eye affected, and associated non-ocular symptoms.
- Past ocular history, (e.g. poor vision in one eye since birth, recurrence of previous disease, particularly inflammatory).
- Past medical history (e.g. for *hypertension* which may be associated with some vascular eye diseases such as central retinal vein occlusion; *diabetes* which may cause retinopathy and systemic *inflammatory* disease such as sarcoid which may also cause ocular inflammation).
- Drug history, since some drugs such as isoniazid and chloroquine may be toxic to the eye.
- Family history (e.g. for ocular diseases known to be inherited such as retinitis pigmentosa, or for disease where family history may be a risk factor, such as glaucoma).
- Presence of allergies.

EXAMINATION

Both structure and function of the eye are examined.

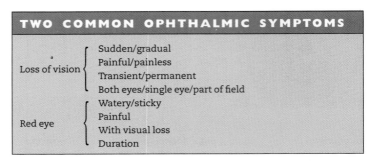

Box 2.1 Two common ophthalmic symptoms and a tree of additional questions that should be asked.

Physiological testing of the eye

VISUAL ACUITY   (Fig. 2.1)

Adults

The standard test of ocular function is the visual acuity. In adults, distance acuity is commonly tested with a Snellen chart read at 6 metres. Going down the chart the size of the letters and their parts decreases from line to line. Increasing acuity implies that the subject is able to resolve the smallest separations. Near vision is tested with a reading test type. The Snellen visual acuity should be measured with the patient wearing distance glasses. If these have been forgotten the patient may view the chart through a pinhole, which will overcome moderate degrees of refractive error.

Children

In children, various methods are used to assess visual acuity, depending on the age of the child:
• Very young children are observed to see if they can follow objects or pick up 'hundreds and thousands' cake decorations.
• The Cardiff Acuity Test can be used to assess vision in one to three year olds. This is a *preferential looking test* based on the finding that children prefer to look at complex rather than plain targets. The grey cards present a variety of figures surrounded by a white band bordered with two black bands. As the width of the bands decreases the picture becomes harder to see against the grey background. The gaze of the child is observed and the examiner estimates whether the object seen is at the top or bottom of the card. When the examiner is unable to identify the position of the

object from the child's gaze it is assumed that the child cannot see the picture.

• Older children are able to identify or match single pictures and letters of varying size (*Sheridan–Gardiner test*).

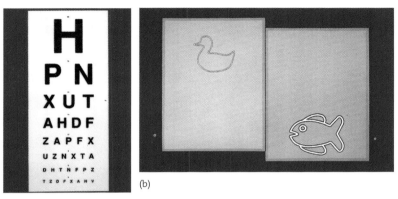

(a)   **Fig. 2.1** Methods of assessing visual acuity: (a) the Snellen chart and (b) examples of Cardiff cards.

VISUAL FIELDS

The visual fields map the peripheral extent of the visual world. Each field can be represented as a series of contours or *isoptres*, demonstrating the ability to resolve a target of given size and brightness. The field is not flat; towards the centre the eye is able to detect much smaller objects than at the periphery. This produces a '*hill of vision*' in which objects which are resolved in finest detail are at the peak of the hill (at the *fovea*) (Fig. 2.2). On the temporal side of the field is the blind spot. This corresponds to the optic nerve head where there is an absence of photoreceptors.

The visual field may be tested in various ways.

CONFRONTATION TESTS

One eye of the patient is covered and the examiner sits opposite closing his eye on the same side. An object, traditionally the head of a large hat pin, is then brought into view from the periphery and moved centrally. The patient is asked to say when he first sees the test object. Each quadrant is tested and the location of the blind spot determined. The patient's field is thus compared to that of the examiner. With practice central *scotomas* (a scotoma is a focal area of decreased sensitivity within the visual field, surrounded by a more sensitive area) can also be identified.

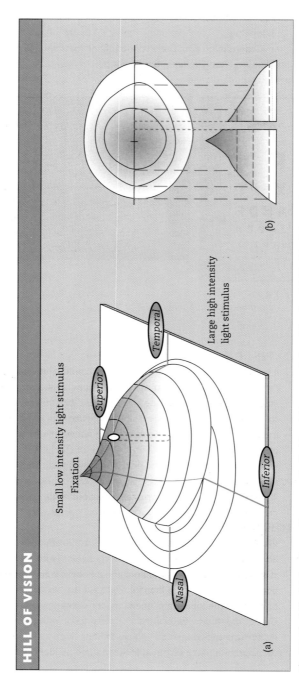

Fig. 2.2 The hill of vision shown diagrammatically (a) and (b) a normal plot of the visual field of the left eye. The different lines (isoptres) correspond to different sizes and intensities of the target. (Adapted with permission from Anderson, D.R. (1982) *Testing the Field of Vision*. Mosby-Year Book, Inc., St Louis.)

Crude testing of the field can be performed as follows:
- Ask the patient to cover one eye. Sit facing the patient and hold up your hands in front of the unoccluded eye, palms facing the patient, one on either side of the midline. Enquire if the two palms apear the same. Repeat the test with the fellow eye. This can be useful in picking up a bitemporal hemianopia (patients may also miss the temporal letters on the Snellen chart when their visual acuity is measured).
- Ask the patient to count the number of fingers which you show in each quadrant of the visual field.

A useful test to identify a neurological field defect is to use a red object. The red field is the most sensitive to optic nerve lesions. A red topped pin is used to perform a confrontation test, the patient being asked to say when he first sees the pin top as red, (not when he first sees the pin top). More simply a red object can be held in each quadrant or hemi-field and the patient asked to compare the quality of red in each location. In a hemianopic field defect the red would appear duller in the affected field.

PERIMETERS

These machines permit more accurate plotting of the visual field. They measure:
- The *kinetic* visual field in which the patient indicates when he first sees a light of a specific size and brightness brought in from the periphery. This is rather like the moving pinhead of the confrontation test.
- The *static* visual field in which the patient indicates when he first sees a stationary light of increasing brightness.

These techniques are particularly useful in chronic ocular and neurological conditions to monitor changes in the visual field (e.g. in glaucoma).

INTRAOCULAR PRESSURE

Intraocular pressure is measured with a Goldmann tonometer (Fig. 2.3). A clear plastic cylinder is pressed against the anaesthetized cornea. The ring of flattening, viewed through the cylinder, is seen as a meniscus made visible by the presence of fluorescein in the tear film (see p. 27). A horizontally disposed prism, within the cylinder, splits the ring of contact into two semicircles. The force applied to the cylinder can be varied to alter the amount of corneal flattening and thus the size of the ring. The force applied can be adjusted so that the two hemicircles just interlock. This is the endpoint of the test, and the force applied, converted into units of ocular pressure (mmHg) can now be read from the tonometer.

Optometrists use a puff of air of varying intensity to produce corneal

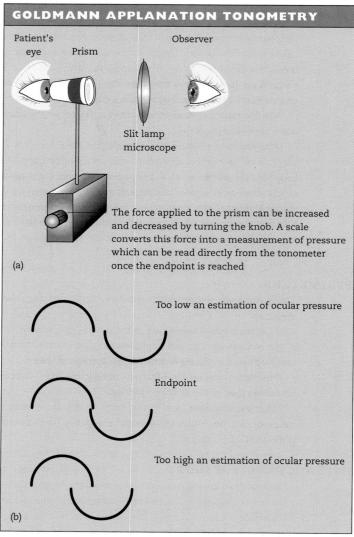

GOLDMANN APPLANATION TONOMETRY

Patient's eye   Prism

Observer

Slit lamp microscope

The force applied to the prism can be increased and decreased by turning the knob. A scale converts this force into a measurement of pressure which can be read directly from the tonometer once the endpoint is reached

(a)

Too low an estimation of ocular pressure

Endpoint

Too high an estimation of ocular pressure

(b)

Fig. 2.3 (a) Measurement of intraocular pressure with a Goldmann tonometer. (b) Two hemicircles are seen by the examiner. The force of contact is increased until the inner borders of the hemicircles just touch. This is the endpoint, at which a fixed amount of flattening of the cornea is achieved.

flattening rather than the prism of the Goldmann tonometer. Various other tonometers are also available including small hand held electronic devices.

PUPILLARY REACTIONS

The size of the pupils (*miosis*, constricted; *mydriasis*, dilated) and their response to light and accommodation gives important information about:
• the function of the afferent pathway controlling the pupils (the optic nerve and tract);
• the function of the efferent pathway.

Examination of the pupils begins with an assessment of the size of the pupils in a uniform light. If there is asymmetry (*anisocoria*) it must be decided whether the small or large pupil is abnormal. A pathologically small pupil (after damage to the sympathetic nervous system) will be more apparent in dim illumination, since dilation of the normal pupil will be greater. A pathologically large pupil (seen in disease of the parasympathetic nervous system) will be more apparent in the light.

Patients with a history of inflammation of the anterior eye (*iritis*), trauma or previous ocular surgery may have structural iris changes which mechanically alter the shape of the pupil (remember the importance of a good history!). Some patients have asymmetrical pupillary diameters unassociated with disease.

In a patient in whom the pupil sizes are equal, the next step is to look for a defect in optic nerve function, using the 'swinging flashlight test'. This is a sensitive index of an afferent conduction defect. The patient is seated in a dimly illuminated room and views a distant object. A torch is directed at each eye in turn while the pupils are observed. A unilateral defect in optic nerve conduction will be demonstrated as a relative afferent pupil defect (RAPD) (see Fig. 2.4).

In order to test the efferent limb of the pupil reflex, the patient is now asked to look at a near object, the normal pupils constrict (in conjunction with accommodation).

EYE MOVEMENTS

These are assessed while sitting facing the patient. Note the following:
• the position of the eyes;
• the range of eye movements;
• the type of eye movements.

An abnormal direction of one of the eyes in the primary position of gaze (looking straight ahead) may suggest a squint. This can be confirmed by performing a cover test (see p. 167).

The range of eye movements is assessed by asking the subject to

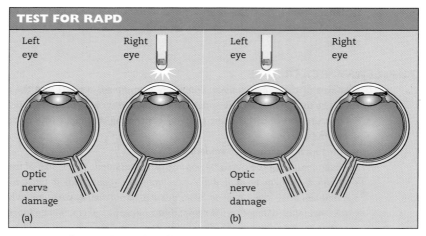

TEST FOR RAPD

Fig. 2.4 The relative afferent pupillary defect. The left optic nerve is damaged. (a) A light shone in the right eye causes both pupils to constrict. (b) When the light is moved to the left eye both pupils dilate because of the lack of afferent drive to the light reflex; a left relative afferent pupillary defect is present. Opacity of the ocular media (e.g. a dense cataract), or damage to the visual pathway beyond the lateral geniculate body will not cause a relative afferent pupillary defect.

follow a moving object. Horizontal, vertical and oblique movements are checked from the primary position of gaze asking the patient to report any double vision (*diplopia*). The presence of oscillating eye movements (*nystagmus*) (see p. 180) is also noted. Movement of the eyes when following an object is recorded. Such movements (*pursuit* movements) are usually smooth but may be altered in disease. The ability to direct gaze rapidly from one object to another (*saccadic* eye movements) can be tested by asking the patient to look at targets (such as the finger) held at either side of the head. These movements should be fast, smooth and accurate (that is they should not overshoot or undershoot the target).

EYELIDS

These are usually at a symmetrical height. The margin of the lid is applied closely to the globe in the healthy eye. If the lid margin is turned away from the globe an *ectropion* is present; if the lid is turned in and the lashes are rubbing against the globe an *entropion* is present.

A drooping lid (*ptosis*) may reflect:
• An anatomical disorder (e.g. a failure of the levator tendon to insert properly into the lid).

- A functional problem (e.g. weakness of the levator muscle in myasthenia gravis).

In assessing ptosis, the distance between the upper and lower lid with the patient looking straight ahead is measured. The excursion of the upper lid from extreme downgaze to extreme upgaze is then recorded. In myasthenia, repeated up and down movement of the lids will increase the ptosis.

Anatomical examination of the eye

LIDS AND ANTERIOR SEGMENT

Simple examination of the eye and adnexae can reveal a great deal about pathological processes within the eye.

EXAMINATION WITHOUT A SLIT LAMP

Without a slit lamp the eye can still be meaningfully examined with a suitable light. Comment can be made on:
- The conjunctiva: is it injected (inflamed), what is the distribution of redness, is a conjunctival haemorrhage present?
- The cornea: is it clear, is there a bright reflection of light from the overlying tear film?
- The anterior chamber: is it intact (if penetrating injury is suspected), is a hypopyon (see p. 89) present?
- The iris and pupil: is the shape of the pupil normal?
- The lens: is there an opacity in the red reflex observed with the ophthalmoscope (see p. 29)?

Box 2.2 Examination of the eye without a slit lamp.

Ophthalmologists use a biomicroscope (*slit lamp*) to examine the eye and lids. This allows the examiner to obtain a magnified stereoscopic view. The slit of light permits a cross-section of the transparent media of the eye to be viewed. By adjusting the angle between this beam and the viewing microscope the light can be used to highlight different structures and pathological processes within the eye. Each structure is carefully examined, starting with the lids and working inwards.

DIAGNOSTIC USE OF FLUORESCEIN

Fluorescein has the property of absorbing light in the blue wavelength and emitting light in the green. The application of fluorescein to the eye can identify corneal abrasions (where the surface epithelial cells have been lost) and leakage of aqueous humour from the eye (Fig. 2.5).

To examine an abrasion:

- a weak solution of the dye is applied to the eye;
- the eye is examined with a blue light;
- the area of the abrasion will appear bright green.

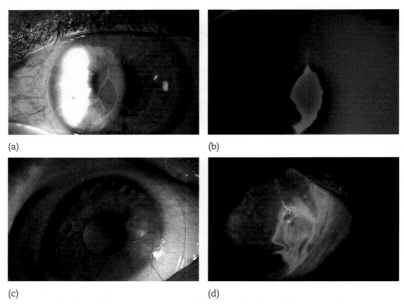

(a)   (b)

(c)   (d)

Fig. 2.5 (a) A corneal abrasion (the corneal epithelial layer has been damaged); (b) fluorescein uniformly stains the area of damage; (c) a perforated cornea leaking aqueous (the leak is protected here with a soft contact lens); (d) the fluorescein fluoresces as it is diluted by the leaking aqueous.

To determine if fluid is leaking from the eye (e.g. after penetrating corneal injury):

- a concentrated 2% solution of fluorescein is applied to the eye;
- the eye is examined with a blue light;
- the dye, diluted by the leaking aqueous, becomes bright green at its junction with the dark fluorescein.

EVERSION OF THE UPPER LID (Fig. 2.6)

The underside of the upper lid is examined by everting it over a small blunt

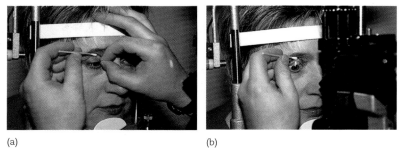

(a)   (b)

Fig. 2.6 Eversion of the upper lid using a cotton bud placed in the lid crease.

ended object (e.g. a cotton bud) placed in the lid crease. This is an important technique to master as foreign bodies may often lodge under the
upper lid causing considerable pain to the victim.

RETINA

The retina is examined by:
- Direct ophthalmoscopy (the conventional ophthalmoscope).
- Indirect ophthalmoscopy, which allows the extremel retinal periphery
to be viewed. The examiner wears a head-mounted binocular microscope
with a light source. A lens placed between the examiner and the eye of the
subject is used to produce an inverted image of the retina (see Fig. 2.7).
  A special contact lens (e.g. a 3-mirror lens) is also used at the slit lamp.
  The latter two techniques are reserved for specialists; the technique
that must be mastered by the non-specialist is direct ophthalmoscopy.
  The direct ophthalmoscope provides:
- an image of the red reflex;
- a magnified view of the optic nerve head, macula, retinal blood vessels
and the retina to the equator.
  It comprises:
- a light source, the size and colour of which can be changed;
- a system of lenses which permits the refractive error of both observer
and patient to be corrected.
  Confident use of the ophthalmoscope comes with practice. The best
results are obtained if the pupil is first dilated with *Tropicamide* a mydriatic
with a short duration of action.
  The patient and examiner must be comfortable and the patient looks
straight ahead at a distant object. The right eye is used to examine the right
eye and the left eye to examine the left eye.
  The examiner, with the ophthalmoscope about 30 cm away from the

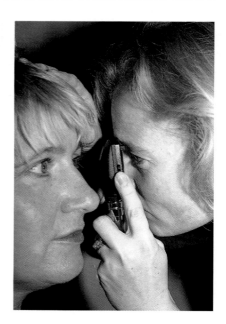

Fig. 2.7 The technique of ophthalmoscopy. Note that the left eye of the observer is used to examine the left eye of the subject. The closer the observer to the patient the larger the field of view.

eye, views the red reflex through the pupil. The correct power of lens in the ophthalmoscope to produce a clear image is found by ratcheting down from a high to a low hypermetropic (plus) correction. Opacities in the cornea or lens of the eye will appear black against the red reflex. The eye is then approached to within a couple of centimetres and the power of the lenses is adjusted in the myopic (minus) direction, to achieve focus on the retina.

The examiner may find it helpful to place a hand on the subject's forehead which can also be used to hold the upper lid open. The retina should now be in view. It is important to try and examine the retina in a logical sequence so that nothing is overlooked.

•   First find the optic disc (Fig. 2.8), assess its margins (are they distinct?), assess the colour of the disc (is it pale?), assess the optic cup (see p. 103).

•   Examine the macular region. Is there a normal foveal reflex (in youth the foveal pit appears as a bright pinpoint of light in the centre of the retina). Are there any abnormal lesions such as haemorrhages, exudates or cotton wool spots?

•   Return to the optic disc and follow each major vessel branch of the vasculature out to the periphery. Are the vessels of normal diameter, do the arteries nip the veins where they cross (*A/V nipping*), are there

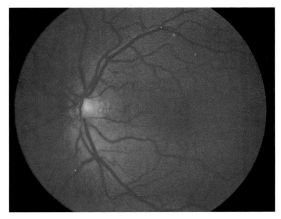

Fig. 2.8 A normal left fundus. Note the optic disc with retinal veins and arteries passing from it to branch over the retina. The large temporal vessels are termed *arcades*. The macula lies temporal to the disc with the fovea at its centre.

any emboli in the arterioles? Also examine the surrounding retina for abnormalities.
- Examine the peripheral retina with a 360° sweep.

DIRECT OPHTHALMOSCOPY

- Use an ophthalmoscope with a good illumination.
- Look at the setting of the ophthalmoscope before examining the patient.
- Retinal examination requires that the examiner is close to the subject. An inadequate view will result if the examiner is too far away.
- Examination through the glasses of a very short-sighted patient may give you a better view.
- Practice, practice, practice.

Box 2.3 Points to watch with direct ophthalmoscopy.

Special examination techniques

DIAGNOSTIC LENSES

Ophthalmologists employ special lenses that can be used in conjunction with the slit lamp to examine particular ocular structures.

A *gonioscopy* lens is a diagnostic contact lens, with a built in mirror that permits visualization of the iridocorneal angle. A larger lens with three mirrors allows the peripheral retina to be seen. Both are applied to the anaesthetized cornea with a lubricating medium. Other lenses can be used to obtain a stereoscopic view of the retina.

RETINOSCOPY

The technique of retinoscopy allows the refractive state of the eye to be measured (i.e. the strength of a corrective spectacle lens). A streak of light from the retinoscope passes into the eye. The reflection from the retina is observed through the retinoscope. By gently moving the retinoscope from side to side the reflected image is seen to move. The direction in which this image moves depends on the refractive error of the eye. By placing trial lenses of differing power in front of the eye the direction in which the reflected image moves is seen to reverse. When this point is reached the refractive error has been determined.

Investigative techniques

ULTRASOUND

This is used extensively in ophthalmology to provide information about the vitreous, retina and posterior coats of the eye, particularly when they cannot be clearly visualized (if, for example, there is a dense cataract or vitreous haemorrhage). Ultrasound is also used to measure the length of the eyeball prior to cataract surgery to estimate the power of the artificial lens that is implanted into the eye (see p. 83).

KERATOMETRY

The shape of the cornea (the radius of curvature) can be measured from the image of a target reflected from its surface. This is important in contact lens assessment, refractive surgery and in calculating the power of an artificial lens implant in cataract surgery.

SYNOPTOPHORE

This machine permits the assessment of binocular single vision, the ability of the two eyes to work together to produce a single image. It is also able to test the range over which the eyes can move away from (*diverge*) or towards each other (*converge*) whilst maintaining a single picture (to measure the range of fusion).

EXOPHTHALMOMETER

This device measures ocular protrusion (*proptosis*).

ELECTROPHYSIOLOGICAL TESTS

The electrical activity of the retina and visual cortex in response to specific visual stimuli, for example a flashing light, can be used to assess the functioning of the retina (*electroretinogram*), RPE (*electro-oculogram*) and the visual pathway (*visually evoked response or potential*).

RADIOLOGICAL IMAGING TECHNIQUES

The CT and MRI scans have largely replaced skull and orbital X-rays in the imaging of the orbit and visual pathway. The newer diagnostic techniques have enhanced the diagnosis of orbital disease (e.g. optic nerve sheath meningioma) and visual pathway lesions such as pituitary tumours. They have also become the first line investigation in orbital trauma.

FLUORESCEIN ANGIOGRAPHY (Fig. 2.9)

This technique provides detailed information about the retinal circulation. Fluorescein dye (see p. 27) is injected into the antecubital vein. A *fundus camera* is used to take photographs of the retina. A blue light is shone into the eye to 'excite' the fluorescein in the retinal circulation. The emitted green light is then photographed through a yellow barrier filter which removes any reflected blue light.

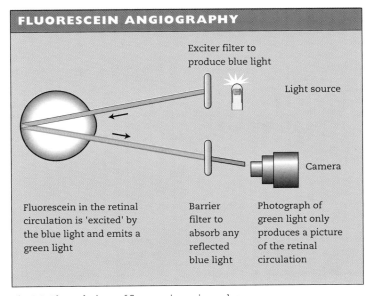

Fig. 2.9 The technique of fluorescein angiography.

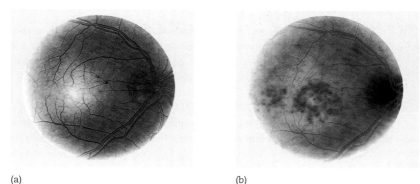

(a)   (b)

Fig. 2.10 A fluorescein angiogram. (a) A photograph of the early phase. The fluorescein in the choroidal circulation can be seen as background fluorescence. (b) In the late phase areas of hyperfluorescence (the dark areas) can be seen around the macula. There has been leakage from abnormal blood vessels into the extravascular tissue space in the macular region (macular oedema).

In this way a fluorescent picture of the retinal circulation is obtained (Fig. 2.10). The dye leaks from abnormal blood vessels (e.g. the new vessels sometimes seen in diabetic eye disease). Areas of ischaemia, due to retinal capillary closure, fail to demonstrate the normal passage of dye (e.g. in a central retinal vein occlusion). The technique is useful both in diagnosis and in planning treatment.

DIGITAL IMAGING AND LASER SCANNING TECHNIQUES

New techniques of retinal imaging are being developed to improve the quality of retinal and optic disc pictures and to permit quantitative assessment of features such as the area of the optic disc and optic disc cup. These will help in the assessment of patients with diseases such as glaucoma and diabetes where the management of these chronic diseases requires an accurate assessment of any change in the disc or retina.

CHAPTER 3

Clinical optics

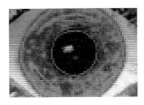

INTRODUCTION

Light can be defined as that part of the electro-magnetic spectrum to which the eye is sensitive. The visible part of the spectrum lies in the waveband of 390 nm to 760 nm. For the eye to generate accurate visual information light must be correctly focused on the retina. The focus must be adjustable to allow equally clear vision of near and distant objects. The cornea, or actually the air/tear interface is responsible for two-thirds and the crystalline lens for one-third of the focusing power of the eye. These two refracting elements in the eye converge the rays of light because:
- The cornea has a higher refractive index than air; the lens has a higher refractive index than the aqueous and vitreous humour that surround it. The velocity of light is reduced in a dense medium so that light is refracted towards the normal. When passing from the air to the cornea or aqueous to lens the rays therefore converge.
- The refracting surface of the cornea and lens are spherically convex.

AMETROPIA

When parallel rays of light from a distant object are brought to focus on the retina with the eye at rest (i.e. not accommodating) the refractive state of the eye is known as *emmetropia* (Fig. 3.1). Such an individual can see sharply in the distance without accommodation.

In *ametropia*, parallel rays of light are not brought to a focus on the retina in an eye at rest. A change in refraction is required to achieve sharp vision.

Ametropia may be divided into:
- *Myopia* (short sight); the optical power of the eye is too high (usually

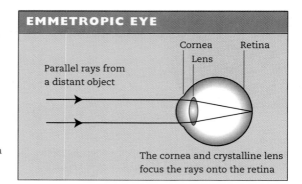

Fig. 3.1 The rays of light in an emmetropic eye are focused on the retina.

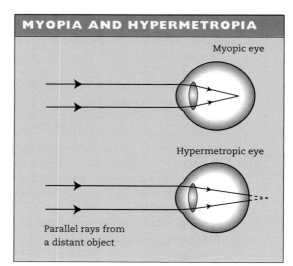

Fig. 3.2 Diagrams demonstrating myopia and hypermetropia.

due to an elongated globe), parallel rays of light are brought to a focus in front of the retina (Fig. 3.2).

• *Hypermetropia* (long sight); the optical power is too low (usually because the eye is too short), parallel rays of light converge towards a point behind the retina.

• *Astigmatism*; the optical power of the cornea in different planes is not equal. Parallel rays of light can never be brought to a point.

All three types of ametropia can be corrected by wearing spectacle lenses. These diverge the rays in myopia, converge the rays in hyperme-

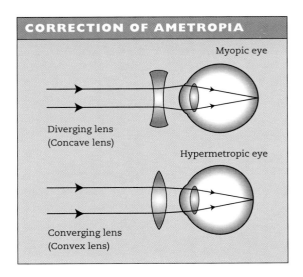

Fig. 3.3 Correction of ametropia with spectacle lenses.

tropia and correct for the nonspherical shape of the cornea in astigmatism (Fig. 3.3). It should be noted that in hypermetropia, accommodative effort will bring distant objects into focus by increasing the power of the lens. This will use up the accommodative reserve for near objects.

ACCOMMODATION AND PRESBYOPIA

As an object is brought nearer to the eye the power of the lens increases, the eyes also converge. This is *accommodation* (Fig. 3.4).

The ability to accommodate decreases with age, reaching a critical point at about 40 when the subject experiences difficulty with near vision (*presbyopia*). This occurs earlier in hypermetropes than myopes. The problem is overcome with convex reading lenses.

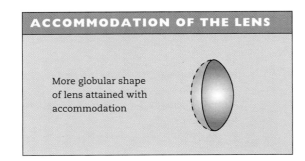

Fig. 3.4 The effect of accommodation on the lens.

OPTICAL CORRECTION AFTER CATARACT EXTRACTION

The lens provides one-third of the refractive power of the eye so that after cataract extraction (the removal of an opaque lens) the eye is rendered highly hypermetropic, a condition termed *aphakia*. This can be corrected by:

* the insertion of an intraocular lens at the time of surgery;
* contact lenses;
* aphakic spectacles.

Intraocular lenses give the best optical results. These mimic the natural lens position. As they are unable to change shape the eye cannot accommodate. An eye with an intraocular lens is said to be *pseudophakic*.

Contact lenses produce slight magnification of the retinal image (110%) but this is not of significance. Insertion, removal and cleaning can be difficult for elderly patients or those with physical disability (arthritis).

Aphakic spectacles have a number of disadvantages:

* They magnify the retinal image by about 133% which causes the patient to misjudge distances. They cannot be used to correct both eyes together if one eye is *phakic* (the natural lens is *in situ*) or pseudophakic because of the disparity in image size. This is termed *aniseikonia* and causes double vision.
* Aphakic lenses induce many optical aberrations including distortion of the image due to the thickness of the lens.

CONTACT LENSES

These are made of plastic materials shaped to sit on the cornea. Different types of material are used to make contact lenses. They are classified as:

* rigid;
* gas permeable;
* soft or hydrophilic.

All contact lenses will retard the diffusion of oxygen to the cornea. Gas permeable lenses are relatively more permeable to oxygen than soft lenses. Although soft lenses are better tolerated, gas permeable lenses have certain advantages:

* their greater oxygen permeability reduces the risk of corneal damage from hypoxia;
* their rigidity allows easier cleaning and offers less risk of infection;

• their rigidity (and that of hard lenses) allows manufacture to correct for astigmatism;

• proteinaceous debris is less likely to adhere to the lens and cause an allergic conjunctivitis.

Gas permeable lenses may be used to correct marked astigmatism. Plane contact lenses may also be used as *bandages*, e.g. in the treatment of some corneal diseases such as a persistent epithelial defect.

SPECTACLES

Spectacles are available to correct most refractive errors. Lenses can be made to correct long and short sight and astigmatism. They are simple and safe to use but may be lost or damaged. Some people find them cosmetically unacceptable and prefer to wear contact lenses. The correction of presbyopia requires additional lens power to overcome the eye's reduced accommodation for near focus. This can be achieved with:

• Separate pairs of glasses for distance and near vision.

• A pair of bifocal lenses where the near correction is added to the lower segment of the distance lens.

• Varifocal lenses where the power of the lens gradually changes from the distance correction (in the upper part) to the near correction (in the lower part). This provides sharper middle-distance vision but the lenses may be difficult to manage.

People with particular needs, such as musicians, may also need glasses for middle distance.

LOW VISION AIDS

Patients with poor vision can be helped by advice on lighting conditions and low vision aids. Clinics specializing in low vision are available in most eye units. Devices used include:

• magnifiers for near vision;

• telescopes for distance vision;

• closed-circuit television to provide magnification and improve contrast;

• large print books;

• talking clocks and watches;

• a variety of gadgets to help the patient manage household tasks.

CHAPTER 4

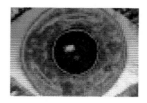

The orbit

INTRODUCTION

The orbit provides:
- protection to the globe;
- attachment which stabilizes the ocular movement;
- transmission of nerves and blood vessels.

Despite the number of different tissues present in the orbit the expression of disease due to different pathologies is often similar.

CLINICAL FEATURES

Proptosis

Proptosis, or *exophthalmos*, is a protrusion of the eye caused by a space-occupying lesion. It can be measured with an exophthalmometer. A difference of more than 3 mm between the two eyes is significant. Various other features give a clue to the pathological process involved (Fig. 4.1).
- If the eye is displaced directly forwards it suggests a lesion that lies within the cone formed by the extraocular muscles. An example would be an optic nerve sheath meningioma.
- If the eye is displaced to one side a lesion outside the muscle cone is likely. For example a tumour of the lacrimal gland displaces the globe to the nasal side.

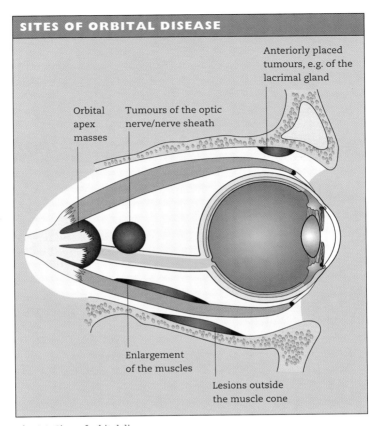

SITES OF ORBITAL DISEASE

Anteriorly placed tumours, e.g. of the lacrimal gland

Orbital apex masses

Tumours of the optic nerve/nerve sheath

Enlargement of the muscles

Lesions outside the muscle cone

Fig. 4.1 Sites of orbital disease.

• A transient proptosis induced by increasing the cephalic venous pressure (by a Valsalva manoeuvre), is a sign of orbital varices.

• The speed of onset of proptosis may also give clues to the aetiology. A slow onset suggests a benign tumour whereas rapid onset is seen in inflammatory disorders, malignant tumours and carotid-cavernous sinus fistula.

• The presence of pain may suggest infection (e.g. orbital cellulitis).

Enophthalmos

Enophthalmos is a backward displacement of the globe. This may be seen following an orbital fracture when orbital contents are displaced into an adjacent sinus. It is also said to occur in Horner's syndrome but this is really a pseudo-enophthalmos due to narrowing of the palpebral fissure. (see p. 145).

Pain

Inflammatory conditions, infective disorders and rapidly progressing tumours cause pain. This is not usually present with benign tumours.

Eyelid and conjunctival changes

Conjunctival injection and swelling suggests an inflammatory or infective process. Infection is associated with reduced eye movements, erythema and swelling of the lids (*orbital cellulitis*). With more anterior lid inflammation (*preseptal cellulitis*) eye movements are full.

Florid engorgement of the conjunctival vessels suggests a vascular lesion caused by the development of a fistula between the carotid artery and the cavernous sinus.

Diplopia

This results from:
• Direct involvement of the muscles in *myositis* and *dysthyroid eye disease*. Movement is restricted in a direction opposite to the field of action of the affected muscle. The eye appears to be tethered (e.g. if the inferior rectus is thickened in thyroid eye disease there will be restriction of upgaze).
• Involvement of the nerve supply to the extraocular muscles. Here diplopia occurs during gaze into the field of action of the muscle (e.g. palsy of the right lateral rectus produces diplopia in right horizontal gaze.

Visual acuity

This may be reduced by:
• exposure keratopathy from severe proptosis, when the cornea is no longer protected by the lids and tear film;
• optic nerve involvement by compression or inflammation;
• distortion of the macula due to compression of the globe by a space occupying lesion.

INVESTIGATION OF ORBITAL DISEASE

The CT and MRI scans have greatly helped in the diagnosis of orbital disease; localising the site of the lesion, demonstrating enlarged intraocular muscles in dysthyroid eye disease and myositis or visualizing fractures to the orbit. Additional systemic tests will be dictated by the differential diagnosis (e.g. tests to determine the primary site of a secondary tumour).

DIFFERENTIAL DIAGNOSIS OF ORBITAL DISEASE

(Traumatic orbital disease is discussed in Chapter 16.)

Disorders of the extraocular muscles

Dysthyroid eye disease and *ocular myositis* present with symptoms and signs of orbital disease. They are described on pp. 174–176.

In children a rapidly developing proptosis may be caused by a *rhabdomyosarcoma* arising from the extraocular muscles.

Infective disorders

Orbital cellulitis is a serious condition which can cause blindness and may spread to cause a brain abscess. The infection often arises from an adjacent ethmoid sinus. The commonest causative organism is Haemophilus Influenzae. The patient presents with:

* a painful eye;
* periorbital inflammation and swelling;
* reduced eye movements;
* conjunctival injection;
* possible visual loss;
* systemic illness and a pyrexia.

An MRI or CT scan are helpful in diagnosis and planning treatment (Fig. 4.2). The condition usually responds to intravenous broad spectrum antibiotics. It may be necessary to drain an abscess or decompress the orbit particularly if the optic nerve is compromised. Optic nerve function must be closely watched, monitoring acuity, colour vision and testing for a relative afferent pupillary defect. Orbital decompression is usually performed with the help of an ENT specialist.

A preseptal cellulitis involves only the lid (Fig. 4.3). It presents with periorbital inflammation and swelling but not the other ocular features of orbital cellulitis.

An orbital mucocoele arises from accumulated secretions within any of the paranasal sinuses when natural drainage of the sinus is blocked. Surgical excision may be required.

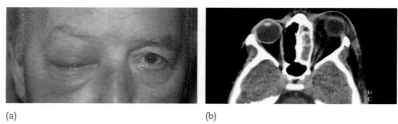

(a)   (b)

Fig. 4.2 (a) The clinical appearance of a patient with right orbital cellulitis. (b) A CT Scan showing a left opaque ethmoid sinus and subperiosteal orbital abscess.

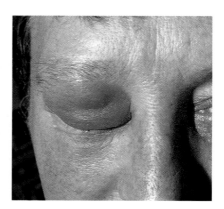

Fig. 4.3 The appearance of a patient with preseptal cellulitis.

Inflammatory disease

The orbit may become involved in various inflammatory disorders including sarcoidosis and orbital pseudotumour, a non-specific lymphofibroblastic disorder. Diagnosis of such conditions is difficult. The presence of other systemic signs of sarcoidosis may be helpful. If an orbital pseudotumour is suspected it may be necessary to biopsy the tissue to differentiate the lesion from a lymphoma.

Vascular abnormalities

A fistula may develop in the cavernous sinus between the carotid artery or a dural artery and the cavernous sinus itself (*carotid-cavernous sinus fistula*). This causes the veins to be exposed to an intravascular high pressure. The eye is proptosed and the conjunctival veins dilated. Extraocular muscle engorgement reduces eye movements and increased pressure in the veins draining the eye causes an increased intraocular pressure. Interventional radiological techniques can be used to close the fistula by embolizing and thrombosing the affected vascular segment.

The orbital veins may become dilated (*orbital varix*) causing intermittent proptosis when venous pressure is raised.

In infants, a *capillary haemangioma* may present as an extensive lesion of the orbit and the surrounding skin (Fig. 4.4). Fortunately most undergo spontaneous resolution in the first 5 years of life. Treatment is indicated if size or position occludes the visual axis and risks the development of amblyopia (see p. 165). Local injection of steroids is usually successful in reducing the size of the lesion.

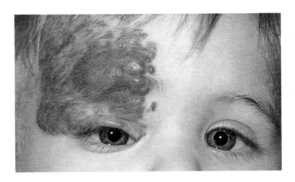

Fig. 4.4 The appearance of a capillary haemangioma.

Orbital tumours (Fig. 4.5)

The following tumours may produce signs of orbital disease.
- lacrimal gland tumours;
- optic nerve gliomas;
- meningiomas;
- lymphomas;
- rhabdomyosarcoma;
- Metastasis from other systemic cancers (neuroblastomas in children, the breast, lung, prostate or gastrointestinal tract in the adult).

A CT or MRI scan will help with the diagnosis. Again systemic investigation, for example to determine the site of a primary tumour, may be required.

Malignant *lacrimal gland tumours* carry a poor prognosis. Benign tumours still require complete excision to prevent malignant transformation. Optic nerve *gliomas* may be associated with *neurofibromatosis*. They

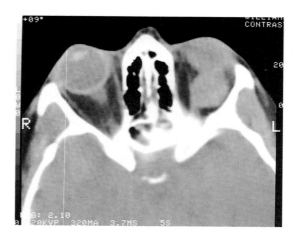

Fig. 4.5 A CT scan showing
a left sided orbital
secondary tumour.

are difficult to treat but are often slow growing and thus may require no intervention. *Meningiomas* of the optic nerve are rare, and may also be difficult to excise. Again they can be observed and some may benefit from treatment with radiotherapy. Meningiomas from the middle cranial fossa may spread through the the optic canal into the orbit. The treatment of *lymphoma* requires a full systemic investigation to determine whether the the lesion is indicative of widespread disease or whether it is localized to the orbit. In the former case the patient is treated with chemotherapy, in the latter with localized radiotherapy.

In children the commonest orbital tumour is a *rhabdomyosarcoma*, a rapidly growing tumour of striated muscle. Chemotherapy is effective if the disease is localized to the orbit.

Dermoid cysts (Fig. 4.6)

These are *teratomas* (epithelial inclusions) which may present in the medial or lateral aspect of the superior orbit. Excision is usually performed for cosmetic reasons.

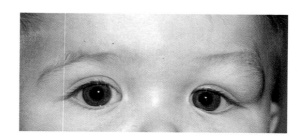

Fig. 4.6 A left dermoid
cyst.

KEY POINTS

- Suspect orbital cellulitis in a patient with periorbital and conjunctival inflammation, particularly if the patient is systemically unwell.
- The commonest cause of bilateral proptosis is dysthyroid disease.
- The commonest cause of unilateral proptosis is also dysthyroid disease.
- Dysthyroid disease may be associated with the serious complications of exposure keratopathy and optic nerve compression.

Box 4.1 Key points in orbital disease.

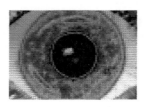

The eyelids

INTRODUCTION

The eyelids are important both in providing physical protection to the eyes and in ensuring a normal tear film and tear drainage. Diseases of the eyelids can be divided into those associated with:

- abnormal lid position;
- inflammation of the lid;
- lid lumps;
- abnormalities of the lashes.

ABNORMALITIES OF LID POSITION

Ptosis (Fig. 5.1)

This is an abnormally low position of the upper eyelid.

PATHOGENESIS

It may be caused by:

I Mechanical factors.

    (a) Large lid lesions pulling down the lid.

    (b) Lid oedema.

(c) Tethering of the lid by conjunctival scarring.

(d) Structural abnormalities including a disinsertion of the aponeurosis of the levator muscle, usually in elderly patients.

2   Neurological factors.

(a) Third nerve palsy (see p. 170).

(b) Horner's syndrome (see p. 145).

(c) Marcus–Gunn jaw-winking syndrome. In this congenital ptosis there is a mis-wiring of the nerve supply to the pterygoid muscle of the jaw and the levator of the eyelid so that the eyelid moves in conjunction with movement of the jaw.

3   Myogenic factors.

(a) Myasthenia gravis (see p. 175).

(b) Some forms of muscular dystrophy.

(c) Chronic external ophthalmoplegia.

SYMPTOMS

Patients present because:

- they object to the cosmetic effect;
- vision may be impaired;
- there are symptoms and signs associated with the underlying cause (e.g. asymmetric pupils in Horner's syndrome, diplopia and reduced eye movements in a third nerve palsy).

SIGNS

There is a reduction in size of the interpalpebral aperture. The upper lid margin, which usually overlaps the upper limbus by 1–2 mm, may be partially covering the pupil. The function of the levator muscle can be tested by measuring the maximum travel of the upper lid from upgaze to downgaze (normally 15–18 mm). Pressure on the brow (frontalis muscle) during this test will prevent its contribution to the lid movement. If myasthenia is suspected the ptosis should be observed during

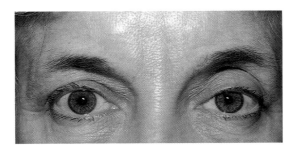

Fig. 5.1 Left ptosis.

repeated lid movement. Increasing ptosis after repeated elevation and depression of the lid is suggestive of myasthenia. Other underlying signs, for example of Horner's syndrome or a third nerve palsy, may be present.

MANAGEMENT

It is important to exclude an underlying cause whose treatment could resolve the problem (e.g. myasthenia gravis). Ptosis otherwise requires surgical correction. In very young children this is usually deferred but may be expedited if pupil cover threatens to induce amblyopia.

Entropion (Fig. 5.2)

This is an inturning, usually of the lower lid. It may occur if the patient looks downwards or be induced by forced lid closure. It is seen most commonly in elderly patients where the orbicularis muscle becomes weakened. It may also be caused by conjunctival scarring distorting the lid (*cicatricial entropion*). The inturned lashes cause irritation of the eye and may also abrade the cornea. The eye may be red. Short-term treatment includes the application of lubricants to the eye or taping of the lid to overcome the inturning. Permanent treatment requires surgery.

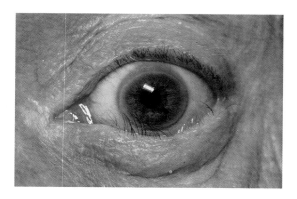

Fig. 5.2 Entropion.

Ectropion (Fig. 5.3)

Here there is an eversion of the lid, usual causes include:
* involutional orbicularis muscle laxity;
* scarring of the periorbital skin;
* seventh nerve palsy.

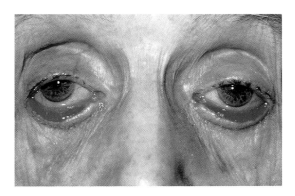

Fig. 5.3 Ectropion.

The malposition of the lids prevents drainage of tears and normal corneal wetting (see p. 58). This again results in an irritable eye. Treatment is again surgical.

INFLAMMATIONS OF THE EYELIDS

Blepharitis (Fig. 5.4)

This is a very common condition of chronic eyelid inflammation. It is sometimes associated with chronic Staphylococcal infection. The condition causes squamous debris, inflammation of the lid margin, skin and eyelash follicles (*anterior blepharitis*). The meibomian glands may be affected independently (meibomian gland disease or *posterior blepharitis*).

SYMPTOMS

These include:
- tired, sore eyes, worse in the morning;
- crusting of the lid margin.

SIGNS

There may be:
- scaling of the lid margins;
- debris in the form of a rosette around the eyelash the base of which may also be ulcerated, a sign of Staphylococcal infection;
- a reduction in the number of eyelashes;
- obstruction and plugging of the meibomian ducts;

- cloudy meibomian secretions;
- injection of the lid margin;
- tear film abnormalities.

In longstanding disease the position of the lid margin may be affected by scarring of the tarsal conjunctiva causing cicatricial entropion.

In severe disease the corneal epithelium is affected (*blepharokeratitis*). Small ulcers may form in the peripheral cornea (*marginal ulceration* secondary to Staphylococcal exotoxins). The conjunctiva becomes injected.

Blepharitis is strongly associated with seborrhoeic dermatitis, atopic eczema and acne rosacea. In rosacea there is hyperaemia and telangiectasia of the facial skin and a rhinophima (a bulbous irregular swelling of the nose with hypertrophy of the sebaceous glands).

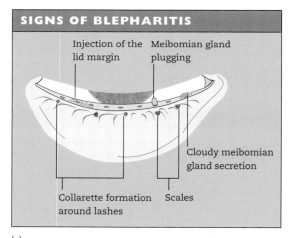

(a)

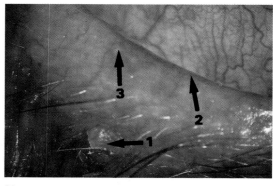

Fig. 5.4 (a) A diagram showing the signs of blepharitis. (b) The clinical appearance of the lid margin. Note (1) the scales on the lashes, (2) dilated blood vessels on the lid margin and (3) plugging of the meibomian glands.

(b)

TREATMENT

This is often difficult. Lid toilet with a cotton bud wetted with bicarbonate solution or diluted baby shampoo helps to remove squamous debris from the eye. Similarly, abnormal meibomian gland secretion can be expressed by lid massage after hot bathing. Staphylococcal lid disease may also require therapy with topical (Fusidic acid gel) and, occasionally, with systemic antibiotics. Meibomian gland function can be improved by oral Tetracycline. Topical steroids may improve an anterior blepharitis but frequent use is best avoided. Posterior blepharitis can be associated with a dry eye which requires treatment with artificial tears.

PROGNOSIS

Although symptoms may be ameliorated by treatment, blepharitis may remain a chronic problem.

BENIGN LID LUMPS AND BUMPS

Chalazion (Fig. 5.5)

This is a common painless condition in which an obstructed meibomian gland causes a granuloma within the tarsal plate. Symptoms are of an unsightly lid swelling which usually resolves within 6 months. If the lesion persists it can be incised and curetted from the conjunctival surface.

An abscess (*internal hordeolum*) may also form within the meibomian gland, which unlike a chalazion is painful. It may respond to topical antibiotics but incision may be necessary.

A stye (*external hordeolum*) is a painful abscess of an eyelash follicle.

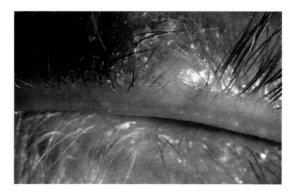

Fig. 5.5 Chalazion.

Treatment requires the removal of the associated eyelash and hot compresses. Most cases are self-limiting. Occasionally systemic antibiotics are required.

Molluscum contagiosum (Fig. 5.6)

This umbilicated lesion found on the lid margin is caused by the pox virus. It causes irritation of the eye. The eye is red and small elevations (follicles) are found on the tarsal conjunctiva. Treatment requires excision of the lesion.

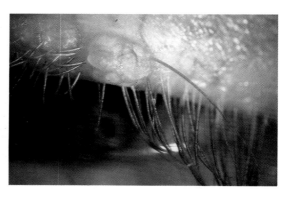

Fig. 5.6 Molluscum contagiosum.

Cysts

Various cysts may form on the eyelids. Sebaceous cysts are opaque. They rarely cause symptoms. They can be excised for cosmetic reasons. A cyst of Moll is a small translucent cyst on the lid margin caused by obstruction of a sweat gland. A cyst of Zeis is an opaque cyst on the eyelid margin caused by blockage of an accessory sebaceous gland. These can be excised for cosmetic reasons.

Squamous cell papilloma

This is a common frond-like lid lesion with a fibrovascular core and thickened squamous epithelium (Fig. 5.7a). It is usually asymptomatic but can be excised for cosmetic reasons with cautery to the base.

Xanthelasmata

These are lipid containing lesions which may be associated with hypercholesterolaemia (Fig. 5.7b). They are excised for cosmetic reasons.

Keratoacanthoma

A brownish pink, fast growing lesion with a central crater filled with keratin Fig. 5.7c. Treatment if required is by excision.

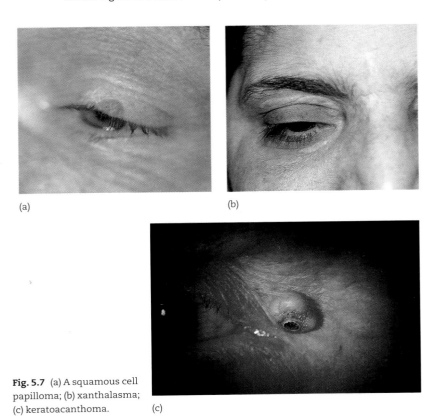

(a)   (b)

(c)

Fig. 5.7 (a) A squamous cell papilloma; (b) xanthalasma; (c) keratoacanthoma.

Naevus (mole)

These lesions are derived from naevus cells (altered melanocytes) and can be pigmented or non-pigmented. No treatment is necessary.

MALIGNANT TUMOURS

Basal cell carcinoma (Fig. 5.8)

This is the most common form of malignant tumour. Ten per cent of cases occur in the eyelids and account for 90% of eyelid malignancy. The tumour is:

- slow growing;
- locally invasive;
- non-metastasising.

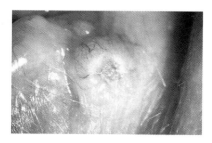

Fig. 5.8 A basal cell carcinoma.

Patients present with a painless lesion on the eyelid which may be nodular, sclerosing or ulcerative (the so-called rodent ulcer). It may have a typical, pale, pearly margin. A high index of suspicion is required. Treatment is by:

- Excision biopsy with a margin of normal tissue surrounding the lesion. Excision may also be controlled with frozen sections when serial histological assessment is used to determine the need for additional tissue removal (Moh's surgery). This minimises destruction of normal tissue.
- Cryotherapy.
- Radiotherapy.

The prognosis is usually very good but deep invasion of the tumour can be difficult to treat.

Squamous cell carcinoma

This is a less common but more malignant tumour which can metastasize to the lymph nodes. It can arise *de novo* or from pre-malignant lesions. It may present as a hard nodule or a scaly patch. Treatment is by excisional biopsy with a margin of healthy tissue.

ABNORMALITIES OF THE LASHES

Trichiasis

This is a common condition in which aberrant eyelashes are directed backwards towards the globe. It is distinct from entropion. The lashes rub against the cornea and cause irritation and abrasion. It may result from any cicatricial process. In developing countries trachoma (see p. 68) is an important cause and trichiasis is an important basis for the associated blindness. Treatment is by epilation of the offending lashes. Recurrence can be treated with cryotherapy or electrolysis. Any underlying abnormality of lid position needs surgical correction.

KEY POINTS

- Blepharitis is a common cause of sore 'tired' irritable eyes.
- A patient with a lid lump and a sore red eye may have molluscum contagiosum.
- Abnormalities of eyelid position can cause corneal disease.

Box 5.1 Key points in eyelid disease.

The lacrimal system

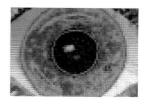

INTRODUCTION

Disorders of the lacrimal system are common and may produce chronic symptoms with a significant morbidity. The lacrimal glands normally produce about 1.2 μl of tears per minute. Some is lost via evaporation. The remainder is drained via the naso-lacrimal system. The tear film is re-formed with every blink.

Abnormalities are found in:
- tear composition;
- the drainage of tears.

ABNORMALITIES IN COMPOSITION

If certain components of the tear film are deficient or there is a disorder of eyelid apposition then there can be a disorder of ocular wetting.

Aqueous insufficiency (Fig. 6.1)

A deficiency of lacrimal secretion occurs with age and results in *keratoconjunctivitis sicca (KCS)* or dry eyes. When this deficiency is associated with a dry mouth and other mucous membranes the condition is called primary *Sjögren's syndrome* (an auto-immune *exocrinopathy*). When KCS is associated with an auto-immune connective tissue disorder the condition is called secondary Sjögren's syndrome. Rheumatoid arthritis is the commonest of these associated disorders.

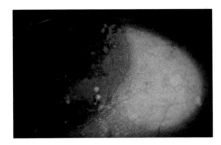

Fig. 6.1 Fluorescein staining of cornea and conjunctiva in a severe dry eye.

SYMPTOMS

Patients have non-specific symptoms of grittiness, burning, photophobia, heaviness of the lids and ocular fatigue. These symptoms are worse in the evening because the eyes dry during the day. In more severe cases visual acuity may be reduced by corneal damage.

SIGNS

In mild cases there are few obvious signs. Staining of the eye with fluorescein will show small dots of fluorescence (*punctate staining*) over the exposed corneal and conjunctival surface. In severe cases tags of abnormal mucus may attach to the corneal surface (*filamentary keratitis*) causing pain due to tugging on these filaments during blinking.

TREATMENT

Supplementation of the tears with tear substitutes helps to reduce symptoms and a humid environment around the eyes can be created with shielded spectacles. In severe cases it may be necessary to occlude the punta with plugs, or more permanently with surgery, to conserve the tears.

PROGNOSIS

Mild disease usually responds to artificial tears. Severe disease such as that in rheumatoid Sjögrens can be very difficult to treat.

Inadequate mucus production

Destruction of the goblet cells occurs in most forms of dry eye, but particularly in Erythema multiforme (Stevens–Johnson's syndrome). There is an acute episode of inflammation causing macular 'target' lesions on the skin and discharging lesions on the eye, mouth and vulva. In the eye this causes conjunctival shrinkage with adhesions forming between the globe and the conjunctiva (*symblepharon*). There may be both an aqueous and mucin deficiency and problems due to lid deformity and trichiasis. Chemical burns of the eye, particularly by alkalis and trachoma, may have a similar end result.

The symptoms are similar to those seen with an aqueous deficiency. Examination may reveal scarred, abnormal conjunctiva and areas of fluorescein staining. Treatment requires the application of artificial lubricants.

Vitamin A deficiency (*xerophthalmia*) is a condition causing childhood blindness on a worldwide scale. It is associated with generalized malnutrition in countries such as India and Pakistan. Goblet cells are lost from the conjunctiva and the ocular surface becomes keratinized (*xerosis*). An aqueous deficiency may also occur. The characteristic corneal melting and perforation which occurs in this condition (*keratomalacia*) may be prevented by early treatment with Vitamin A.

Abnormal or inadequate production of meibomian oil

Absence of the oil layer causes tear film instability, associated with blepharitis (see p. 51).

Malposition of the eyelid margins

If the lid is not apposed to the eye (*ectropion*), or there is insufficient closure of the eyes (e.g. in a seventh nerve palsy or if the eye protrudes

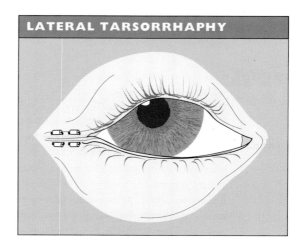

LATERAL TARSORRHAPHY

Fig. 6.2 A tarsorrhaphy protects a previously exposed cornea.

(*proptosis*) as in dysthyroid eye disease) the preocular tear film will not form adequately. Correction of the lid deformity is the best answer to the problem. If the defect is temporary, artificial tears and lubricants can be applied. If lid closure is inadequate a temporary ptosis can be induced with a local injection of Botulinum toxin into the levator muscle. A more permanent result can be obtained by suturing together part of the apposed margins of the upper and lower lids (e.g. *lateral tarsorrhaphy*; Fig. 6.2).

DISORDERS OF TEAR DRAINAGE

When tear production exceeds the capacity of the drainage system, excess tears overflow onto the cheeks. It may be caused by:
- irritation of the ocular surface, e.g. by a corneal foreign body or infection;
- occlusion of any part of the drainage system (when the tearing is termed *epiphora*).

Obstruction of tear drainage (infant)

The naso-lacrimal system develops as a solid cord which subsequently canalises and is patent just before term. Congenital obstruction of the duct is common. The distal end of the naso-lacrimal duct may remain imperforate, causing a watering eye. If the canaliculi also become partly obstructed the non-draining pool of tears in the sac may become infected and accumulate as a *mucocele* or cause *dacrocystitis*. Diagnostically the discharge may be expressed from the puncta by pressure over the lacrimal sac. The conjunctiva, however, is not inflamed. Most obstructions resolve spontaneously in the first year of life. If epiphora persists beyond this time, patency can be achieved by passing a probe via the punctum through the naso-lacrimal duct to perforate the occluding membrane (*probing*). A general anaesthetic is required.

Obstruction of tear drainage (adult)

The tear drainage system may become blocked at any point, although the most common site is the nasolacrimal duct. Causes include infection or direct trauma to the nasolacrimal system.

HISTORY

The patient complains of a watering eye sometimes associated with stickiness. The eye is white. Symptoms may be worse in the wind or in cold weather. There may be a history of previous trauma or infection.

SIGNS

A stenosed punctum may be apparent on slit lamp examination. Epiphora is unusual if one punctum continues to drain. Acquired obstruction beyond the punctum is diagnosed by syringing the naso-lacrimal system with saline using a fine cannula inserted into a canaliculus. A patent system is indicated when the patient tastes the saline as it reaches the pharynx. If there is an obstruction of the nasolacrimal duct then fluid will regurgitate from the non-canulated punctum. The exact location of the obstruction can be confirmed by injecting a radio-opaque dye into the naso-lacrimal system (*dacrocystogram*); X-rays are then used to follow the passage of the dye through the system.

TREATMENT

It is important to exclude other ocular disease that may contribute to watering such as blepharitis. Repair of the occluded nasolacrimal duct requires surgery to connect the mucosal surface of the lacrimal sac to the nasal mucosa by removing the intervening bone (*dacrocystorhinostomy or DCR* (Fig. 6.3)). The operation is usually performed through an incision on the side of the nose but it may also be performed endoscopically through the nasal passages.

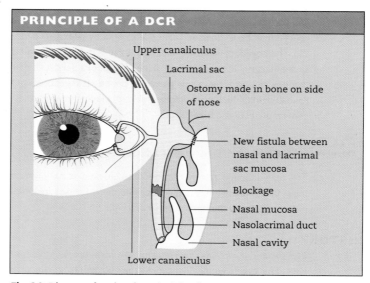

PRINCIPLE OF A DCR

Upper canaliculus
Lacrimal sac
Ostomy made in bone on side of nose
New fistula between nasal and lacrimal sac mucosa
Blockage
Nasal mucosa
Nasolacrimal duct
Nasal cavity
Lower canaliculus

Fig. 6.3 Diagram showing the principle of a DCR.

INFECTIONS OF THE NASO-LACRIMAL SYSTEM

Closed obstruction of the drainage system predisposes to infection of the sac (*dacryocystitis*; Fig. 6.4). The organism involved is usually Staphylococcus. Patients present with a painful swelling on the medial side of the orbit, which is the enlarged, infected sac. Treatment is with systemic antibiotics. A *mucocoele* results from a collection of mucus in an obstructed sac, it is not infected. In either case a DCR may be necessary to prevent recurrence.

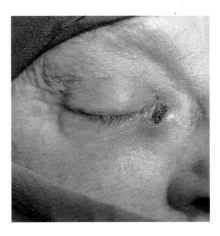

Fig. 6.4 Dacrocystitis, unusually, in this case, pointing through the skin.

KEY POINTS

- Dry eyes can cause significant ocular symptoms and signs.
- A watery eye in a newborn child is commonly due to non-patency of the nasolacrimal duct. Most spontaneously resolve within the first year of life.

Box 6.1 Key points in lacrimal disease.

CHAPTER 7

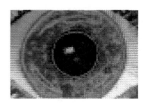

Conjunctiva, cornea and sclera

INTRODUCTION

Disorders of the conjunctiva and cornea are a common cause of symptoms. The ocular surface is regularly exposed to the external environment and subject to trauma, infection and allergic reactions which account for the majority of diseases in these tissues. Degenerative and structural abnormalities account for a minority.

Symptoms

Patients may complain of the following:

1 Pain and irritation. Conjunctivitis is seldom associated with anything more than mild discomfort. Pain signifies something more serious such as corneal injury or infection. This symptom helps differentiate conjunctivitis from corneal disease.

2 Redness. In conjunctivitis the entire conjunctival surface including that covering the tarsal plates is involved. If the redness is localized to the limbus the following should be considered:

  (a) keratitis (an inflammation of the cornea);
  (b) uveitis;
  (c) acute glaucoma.

3 Discharge. Purulent discharge suggests a bacterial conjunctivitis. Viral conjunctivitis is associated mainly with a watery discharge.

4 Visual loss. This occurs only when the central cornea is affected. Loss of vision is thus an important symptom requiring urgent action.

5 Patients with corneal disease may also complain of photophobia.

Signs

The following features may be seen in conjunctival disease:

- Papillae. These are raised lesions on the upper tarsal conjunctiva, about 1 mm in diameter with a central vascular core. They are non-specific signs of chronic inflammation. They result from fibrous septa between the conjunctiva and subconjunctiva which allow only the intervening tissue to swell with inflammatory infiltrate. *Giant papillae*, found in allergic eye disease, are formed by the coalescence of papillae (see Fig. 7.4).

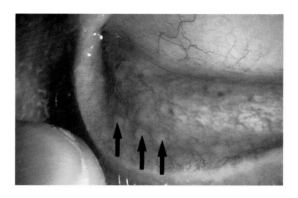

Fig. 7.1 The clinical appearance of follicles.

- Follicles (Fig. 7.1). These are raised, gelatinous, oval lesions about 1 mm in diameter found usually in the lower tarsal conjunctiva and occasionally at the limbus. Each follicle represents a lymphoid collection with its own germinal centre. Unlike papillae, the causes of follicles are more specific (e.g. viral and chlamydial infections).
- Dilation of the conjunctival vasculature (termed 'injection').
- Subconjunctival haemorrhage, often bright red in colour because it is fully oxygenated by the ambient air, through the conjunctiva.

The features of corneal disease are different and include the following:
- Epithelial and stromal oedema may develop causing clouding of the cornea.
- Cellular infiltrate in the stroma causing focal granular white spots.
- Deposits of cells on the corneal endothelium (termed *keratic precipitates* or *KPs* usually lymphocytes or macrophages, see p. 89).
- Chronic keratitis may stimulate new blood vessels superficially, under the epithelium (*pannus*; Fig. 7.2) or deeper in the stroma. Stromal oedema, which causes swelling and separates the collagen lamellae, facilitates vessel invasion.

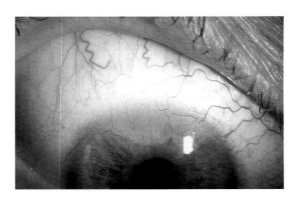

Fig. 7.2 Pannus.

- Epithelial erosions are punctate or more extensive patches of epithelial loss which are best detected using fluorescein dye viewed with blue illumination.

CONJUNCTIVA

Inflammatory diseases of the conjunctiva

BACTERIAL CONJUNCTIVITIS

Patients present with:
- redness of the eye;
- discharge;
- ocular irritation.

The commonest causative organisms are Staphylococcus, Streptococcus, Pneumococcus and Haemophilus. The condition is usually self-limiting although a broad spectrum antibiotic eye drop will hasten resolution. Conjunctival swabs for culture are indicated if the condition fails to resolve.

ANTIBIOTICS

Ceftazidine
Chloramphenicol
Ciprofloxacin
Fusidic acid
Gentamicin
Neomycin
Ofloxacin
Tetracycline

Box. 7.1 Some of the antibiotics available for topical ophthalmic use. Chloramphenicol is an effective broad spectrum agent, a small risk of bone marrow aplasia is a moot point.

Ophthalmia neonatorum, which refers to any conjunctivitis that occurs in the neonatal period (first 28 days of life), is a notifiable disease. Swabs for culture are mandatory. It is also important that the cornea is examined to exclude any ulceration.

The commonest organisms are:

- Bacterial conjunctivitis (usually Gram positive).
- *Neisseria gonorrhoea.* In severe cases this can cause corneal perforation. Penicillin given topically and systemically is used to treat the local and systemic disease respectively.
- Herpes simplex, which can cause corneal scarring. Topical antivirals are used to treat the condition.
- Chlamydia. This may be responsible for a chronic conjunctivitis and cause sight threatening corneal scarring. Topical tetracycline ointment and systemic erythromycin is used is used to treat the local and systemic disease respectively.

VIRAL CONJUNCTIVITIS

This is distinguished from bacterial conjunctivitis by:

- a watery and limited purulent discharge;
- the presence of conjunctival follicles and enlarged pre-auricular lymph nodes;
- there may also be lid oedema and excessive lacrimation.

The conjunctivitis is self-limiting but highly contagious. The commonest causative agent is Adenovirus and to a lesser extent Coxsackie and Picornavirus. Adenoviruses can also cause a conjunctivitis associated with the formation of a pseudomembrane across the conjunctiva. Certain adenovirus serotypes also cause a troublesome punctate keratitis. Treatment for the conjunctivitis is unnecessary unless there is a secondary bacterial infection. Patients must be given hygiene instruction to minimize the spread of infection (e.g. using separate towels). Treatment of keratitis is controversial. The use of topical steroids damps down symptoms and causes corneal opacities to resolve but rebound inflammation is common when the steroid is stopped.

CHLAMYDIAL INFECTIONS

Different serotypes of the obligate intracellular organism Chlamydia trachomatis are responsible for two forms of ocular infections.

Inclusion keratoconjunctivitis

This is a sexually transmitted disease and may take a chronic course (up to 18 months) unless adequately treated. Patients present with a mucopurulent follicular conjunctivitis and develop a micropannus (peripheral corneal vascularization and scarring) associated with subepithelial scarring. Urethritis or cervicitis is common. Diagnosis is confirmed by detection of chlamydial antigens, using immunofluorescence, or by identification of typical inclusion bodies by Giemsa staining in conjunctival swab or scrape specimens.

Inclusion conjunctivitis is treated with topical and systemic tetracycline. The patient should be referred to a sexually transmitted diseases clinic.

Trachoma (Fig. 7.3)

This is the commonest infective cause of blindness in the world although it is uncommon in developed countries. The housefly acts as a vector and the disease is encouraged by poor hygiene and overcrowding in a dry, hot climate. The hallmark of the disease is subconjunctival fibrosis caused by frequent re-infections associated with the unhygienic conditions. Blindness may occur due to corneal scarring from recurrent keratitis and trichiasis.

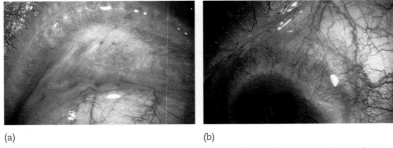

(a)   (b)

Fig. 7.3 Scarring of (a) the upper lid (inverted) and (b) the cornea in trachoma.

Trachoma is treated with oral or topical tetracycline or erythromycin. Azithromycin, an alternative, requires only one application. Entropion and trichiasis require surgical correction.

ALLERGIC CONJUNCTIVITIS

This may be divided into acute and chronic forms:

1   Acute (hayfever conjunctivitis). This is an acute IgE mediated reaction to airborne allergens (usually pollens). Symptoms and signs include:
    (a) itchiness;
    (b) conjunctival injection and swelling (chemosis);
    (c) lacrimation.
2   Vernal conjunctivitis (spring catarrh) is also mediated by IgE. It often

affects male children with a history of atopy. It may be present all year long. Symptoms and signs include:

(a) itchiness;

(b) photophobia;

(c) lacrimation;

(d) papillary conjunctivitis (papillae may coalesce to form giant cobblestones; Fig. 7.4);

(e) focal infiltrates (white spots) at the limbus;

(f) punctate lesions on the corneal epithelium;

(g) an opaque plaque which in severe disease replaces an oval upper zone of the corneal epithelium.

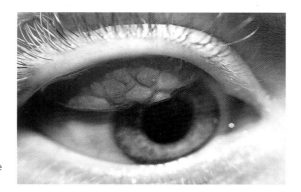

Fig. 7.4 The appearance of giant (cobblestone) papillae in vernal conjunctivitis.

Initial therapy is with antihistamines and mast cell stabilizers (e.g. sodium cromoglycate; nodocromyl; lodoxamide). Topical steroids are required in severe cases but long-term use is avoided if possible because of the possibility of steroid induced glaucoma or cataract.

Contact lens wearers may develop an allergic reaction to their lenses or to lens cleaning materials leading to a *giant papillary conjunctivitis (GPC)* with a mucoid discharge. Whilst this may respond to topical treatment with mast cell stabilizers it is often necessary to stop lens wear for a period or even permanently. Some patients are unable to continue contact lens wear due to recurrence of the symptoms.

Conjunctival degenerations

Cysts are common in the conjunctiva. They rarely cause symptoms but if necessary can be removed.

Pingueculae and *pterygia* are found on the interpalpebral bulbar conjunctiva. They are thought to result from excessive exposure to the reflected or direct ultraviolet component of sunlight. Histologically the cottagen structure is altered. Pingueculae are yellowish lesions that never impinge on the cornea, pterygia are wing shaped and located nasally, with the apex towards the cornea onto which they progressively extend (Fig. 7.5). They may cause irritation and, if extensive, may encroach onto the visual axis. They can be excised but may recur.

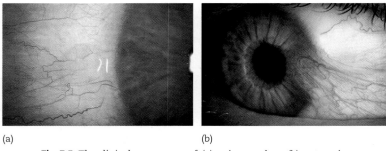

(a)   (b)

Fig. 7.5 The clinical appearance of: (a) a pingueculum; (b) a pterygium.

CONJUNCTIVAL TUMOURS

These are rare. They include:

• Squamous cell carcinoma. An irregular raised area of conjunctiva which may invade the deeper tissues.

• Malignant melanoma. The differential diagnosis from benign pigmented lesions (for example a naevus) may be difficult. Review is necessary to assess whether the lesion is increasing in size. Biopsy to achieve a definitive diagnosis, may be required.

CORNEA

Infective corneal lesions

HERPES SIMPLEX KERATITIS

Type 1 Herpes simplex (HSV) is a common and important cause of ocular disease. Type 2 which causes genital disease may occasionally cause keratitis and infantile chorioretinitis. Primary infection by HSV1 is usually acquired early in life by close contact such as kissing. It is accompanied by:

• fever;

• vesicular lid lesions;

• follicular conjunctivitis;

- pre-auricular lymphadenopathy;
- some cases may be asymptomatic.

The cornea may not be involved although punctate epithelial damage may be seen. Recurrent infection results from activation of a virus lying latent in the trigeminal ganglion of the fifth cranial nerve. The virus travels in the nerve to the eye. This often occurs if the patient is debilitated for some reason (e.g. psychiatric disease, systemic illness, immunosuppression). It is characterized by the appearance of *dendritic ulcers* on the cornea (Fig. 7.6). These usually heal without a scar. If the stroma is also involved oedema develops causing a loss of corneal transparency. Involvement of the stroma may lead to permanent scarring. If corneal scarring is severe a corneal graft may be required to restore vision. Uveitis and glaucoma may accompany the disease. *Disciform keratitis* is an immunogenic reaction to herpes antigen in the stroma and presents as stromal clouding without ulceration, often associated with iritis.

Dendritic lesions are treated with topical antivirals which typically heal within 2 weeks. Topical steroids must not be given to patients with a dendritic ulcer since they may cause extensive corneal ulceration. In patients with stromal involvement (keratitis) steroids are used under ophthalmic supervision and with antiviral cover.

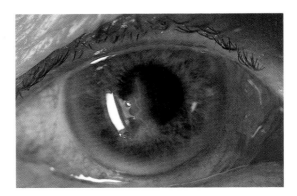

Fig. 7.6 A dendritic ulcer seen in Herpes simplex infection.

Box 7.2 Some of the topical antiviral agents available for ocular therapy.

ANTIVIRAL AGENTS
Idoxuridine
Vidarabine
Trifluorothymidine
Acyclovir

HERPES ZOSTER OPHTHALMICUS
(OPHTHALMIC SHINGLES) (Fig. 7.7)

This is caused by the Varicella-zoster virus which is responsible for chickenpox. The ophthalmic division of the trigeminal nerve is affected. Unlike Herpes simplex infection there is usually a prodromal period with the patient systemically unwell. Ocular manifestations are usually preceded by the appearance of vesicles in the distribution of the ophthalmic division of the trigeminal nerve. Ocular problems are more likely if the naso-ciliary branch of the nerve is involved (vesicles at the root of the nose).

Signs include:
- lid swelling (which may be bilateral);
- keratitis;
- iritis;
- secondary glaucoma.

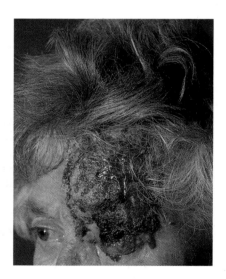

Fig. 7.7 The clinical appearance of Herpes zoster ophthalmicus.

Reactivation of the disease is often linked to unrelated systemic illness. Oral antiviral treatment (e.g. acyclovir) is effective in reducing post-infective neuralgia (a severe chronic pain in the area of the rash) if given within 3 days of the skin vesicles erupting. Ocular disease may require treatment with topical antivirals and steroids.

The prognosis of herpetic eye disease has improved since antiviral treatment became available. Both simplex and zoster cause anaesthesia of the cornea. Non-healing indolent ulcers may be seen following simplex infection and are difficult to treat.

BACTERIAL KERATITIS

Pathogenesis
A host of bacteria may infect the cornea.

Box 7.3 Some of the bacteria responsible for corneal infection.

> **BACTERIA OF CORNEAL INFECTION**
>
> - Staphylococcus epidermidis
> - Staphylococcus aureus.
> - Streptococcus pneumoniae.
> - Coliforms.
> - Pseudomonas.
> - Haemophilus.

All can be found in the conjunctival sac as part of the normal flora. The conjunctiva and cornea are protected against infection by:
- blinking;
- washing away of debris by the flow of tears;
- entrapment of foreign particles by mucus;
- the antibacterial properties of the tears;
- the barrier function of the corneal epithelium (Neisseria Gonnorrhoea is the only organism that can penetrate the intact epithelium).

Predisposing causes of bacterial keratitis include:
- keratoconjunctivitis sicca (dry eye);
- a breach in the corneal epithelium (e.g. following trauma);
- contact lens wear;
- prolonged use of topical steroids.

Symptoms and signs
These include:
- pain, usually severe unless the cornea is anaesthetic;
- purulent discharge;
- ciliary injection;
- visual impairment (severe if the visual axis is involved);
- hypopyon sometimes (a mass of white cells collected in the anterior chamber; see pp. 89–90);
- a white corneal opacity which can often be seen with the naked eye (Fig. 7.8).

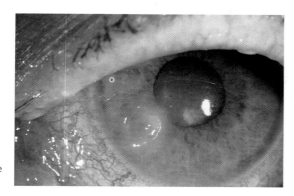

Fig. 7.8 Clinical appearance of a corneal ulcer.

Treatment

Scrapes are taken from the base of the ulcer for Gram staining and culture. The patient is then treated with intensive topical antibiotics often with dual therapy (e.g. cefuroxime against Gram +ve bacteria and gentamicin for Gram −ve bacteria) to cover most organisms. The drops are given hourly day and night for the first couple of days and reduced in frequency as clinical improvement occurs. In severe or unresponsive disease the cornea may perforate. This can be treated initially with tissue adhesives (cyano-acrylate glue) and a subsequent corneal graft. A persistent scar may also require a corneal graft to restore vision.

ACANTHAMOEBA KERATITIS (Fig. 7.9)

This freshwater amoeba is responsible for infective keratitis. The infection is becoming more common due to the increasing use of contact lenses. A painful keratitis with prominence of the corneal nerves results. The amoeba can be isolated from the cornea (and from the contact lens case)

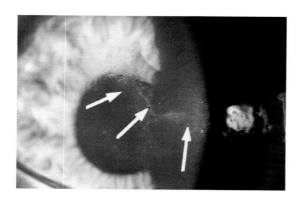

Fig. 7.9 The clinical appearance of acanthamoeba keratitis. Arrows indicate neurokeratitis.

with a scrape and cultured on special plates impregnated with Escherichia coli. Topical chlorhexidine, polyhexamethylene biguanide (PHMB) and propamidine are used to treat the condition.

FUNGAL KERATITIS

This is unusual in the UK but more common in warmer climates such as the southern USA. In India it accounts for 30–50% of infective keratitis. It should be considered in:

- lack of response to antibacterial therapy in corneal ulceration;
- cases of trauma with vegetable matter;
- cases associated with the prolonged use of steroids.

The corneal opacity appears fluffy and satellite lesions may be present. Liquid and solid Sabaroud's media are used to grow the fungi. Incubation may need to be prolonged. Treatment requires topical antifungal drops such as Pimaricin 5%.

INTERSTIAL KERATITIS

This term is used for any keratitis that affects the corneal stroma without epithelial involvement. Classically the most common cause was syphillis, leaving a mid stromal scar with the outline ('ghost') of blood vessels seen. Corneal grafting may be required when the opacity is marked and visual acuity reduced.

Corneal dystrophies (Fig. 7.10)

These are rare inherited disorders. They affect different layers of the cornea and often affect corneal transparency. They may be divided into:

- Anterior dystrophies involving the epithelium. These may present with recurrent corneal erosion.

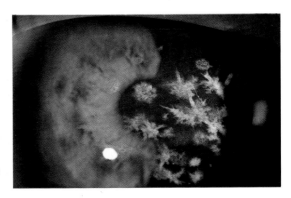

Fig. 7.10 Example of a corneal dystrophy (granular dystrophy).

- Stromal dystrophies presenting with visual loss. If very anterior they may cause corneal erosion and pain.
- Posterior dystrophies which affect the endothelium and cause gradual loss of vision due to oedema. They may also cause pain due to epithelial erosion.

Disorders of shape

KERATOCONUS

This is usually a sporadic disorder but may occasionally be inherited. Thinning of the centre of the cornea leads to a conical corneal distortion. Vision is affected but there is no pain. Initially the associated astigmatism can be corrected with glasses or contact lenses. In severe cases a corneal graft may be required.

Central corneal degenerations

BAND KERATOPATHY (Fig. 7.11)

Band keratopathy is the subepithelial deposition of calcium phosphate in the exposed part of the cornea where CO_2 loss and the consequent raised pH favour its deposition. It is seen in eyes with chronic uveitis or glaucoma and may cause visual loss or discomfort if epithelial erosions form over the band. If symptomatic it can be scraped off aided by a chelating agent such as sodium edetate. The excimer laser can also be effective in treating these patients by ablating the affected cornea. Band keratopathy

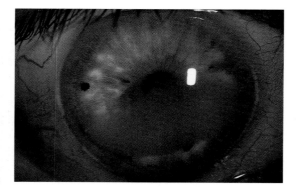

Fig. 7.11 Band keratopathy.

can also be a sign of systemic hypercalcaemia as in hyperparathyroidism or renal failure. The lesion is then more likely to occupy the 3 O'clock and 9 O'clock positions of the limbal cornea.

Peripheral corneal degenerations

CORNEAL THINNING

A rare cause of painful peripheral corneal thinning is *Mooren's ulcer*, a condition with an immune basis. Corneal thinning or melting can also be seen in collagen diseases such as rheumatoid arthritis and Wegeners granulomatosis. Treatment can be difficult and both sets of disorder require systemic and topical immunosuppression. Where there is an associated dry eye it is important to ensure adequate corneal wetting and corneal protection (see p. 59).

LIPID ARCUS

This is a peripheral white ring-shaped lipid deposit, separated from the limbus by a clear interval. It is most often seen in normal elderly people (*arcus senilis*) but in young patients it may be a sign of hyperlipidaemia. No treatment is required.

Corneal grafting (Fig. 7.12)

Donor corneal tissue can be grafted into a host cornea to restore corneal clarity or repair a perforation. Donor corneae can be stored and are banked so that corneal grafts can be performed on routine operating lists.

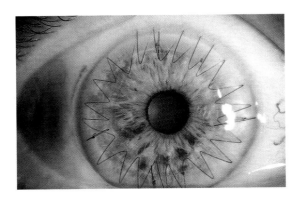

Fig. 7.12 A corneal graft, note the interrupted and the continuous sutures at the interface between graft and host.

The avascular host cornea provides an immune privileged site for grafting, with a high success rate. Tissue can be HLA-typed for grafting of vascularized corneae at high risk of immune rejection. The patient uses steroid eye drops for some time after the operation to prevent graft rejection. Complications such as astigmatism can be dealt with surgically or by suture adjustment.

GRAFT REJECTION

Any patient who has had a corneal graft and who complains of redness, pain or visual loss must be seen urgently by an eye specialist, as this may indicate graft rejection. Examination shows graft oedema, iritis and a line of activated T-cells attacking the graft endothelium. Intensive topical steroid application in the early stages can restore graft clarity.

Refractive surgery

The refractive power of the cornea, the first refractive element of the eye, can be surgically modified to correct any refractive error. Radial keratotomy (RK) is used to correct short-sightedness and involves the placement of radial incisions in the peripheral cornea to flatten the central region and reduce its optical power. The procedure has to some extent been replaced by a laser technique, photorefractive keratoplasty (PRK). Following the removal of the corneal epithelium, the shape of the anterior corneal stroma is remodelled by ablating the superficial stroma with a laser. The exact amount of cornea to be removed depends on the refractive error to be corrected. Myopia, hypermetropia and to a lesser extent astigmatism can all be dealt with.

The major problems with refractive surgery are:
- under or over correction;
- regression of the correction towards the initial refractive error;
- glare when driving at night;
- fluctuating vision.

SCLERA

EPISCLERITIS

This inflammation of the superficial layer of the sclera causes mild discomfort. It is rarely associated with systemic disease. It is usually self-limiting but as symptoms are tiresome, topical anti-inflammatory treatment can be given. In rare, severe disease, systemic non-steroidal anti-inflammatory treatment may be helpful.

SCLERITIS (Fig. 7.13)

This is a more severe condition than episcleritis and may be associated with the collagen-vascular diseases, most commonly rheumatoid arthritis. It is a cause of intense ocular pain. Both inflammatory areas and ischaemic areas of the sclera may occur. Characteristically the affected sclera is swollen. The following may complicate the condition:

- scleral thinning (*scleromalacia*), sometimes with perforation;
- keratitis;
- uveitis;
- cataract formation;
- glaucoma.

Treatment may require high doses of systemic steroids or in severe cases cytotoxic therapy and investigation to find any associated systemic disease.

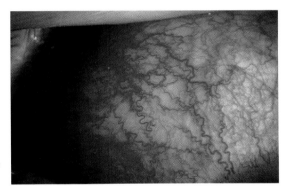

Fig. 7.13 The appearance of scleritis.

Scleritis affecting the posterior part of the globe may cause choroidal effusions or simulate a tumour.

KEY POINTS

- Avoid the unsupervised use of topical steroids in treating ophthalmic conditions since complications may be serious.
- In contact lens wearers a painful red eye is serious, it may imply an infective keratitis.

Box 7.4 Key points in corneal disease.

The lens and cataract

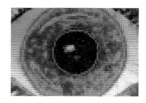

INTRODUCTION

The lens is biconvex and transparent. It is held in position behind the iris by the suspensory ligament whose zonular fibres are composed of the protein fibrillin which attach its equator to the ciliary body. Disease may affect structure, shape and position.

CHANGE IN LENS STRUCTURE

Cataract

Opacification of the lens of the eye (*cataract*) is the commonest cause of treatable blindness in the world. The large majority of cataracts occur in older age as a result of the cumulative exposure to environmental and other influences such as smoking, UV light and blood sugar levels. This is sometimes referred to as *age-related cataract*. A smaller number are associated with specific ocular or systemic disease and defined physico-chemical mechanisms.

OCULAR CONDITIONS

Trauma
Uveitis
High myopia
Topical medication (particularly steroid eye drops).
Intraocular tumour

Box 8.1 Ocular conditions associated with cataract.

SYSTEMIC CAUSES
Diabetes
Other metabolic disorders (including galactosaemia, Fabry's disease, hypocalcaemia)
Systemic drugs (particularly steroids, chlorpromazine)
Infection (congenital rubella)
Myotonic dystrophy
Atopic dermatitis
Systemic syndromes (Down's, Lowe's)
Congenital (inherited) cataract
X-radiation

Box 8.2 Systemic causes of cataract.

SYMPTOMS

An opacity in the lens of the eye:

- causes a painless loss of vision;
- causes glare;
- may change refractive error;

In infants, cataract may cause amblyopia (a failure of normal visual development) because the retina is deprived of a formed image. Infants with suspected cataract or a family history of congenital cataracts should be seen as a matter of urgency by an ophthalmologist (see p. 86).

SIGNS

Visual acuity is reduced. In some patients the acuity measured in a dark room may seem satisfactory, whereas if the same test is carried out in bright light or sunlight the acuity will be seen to fall, as a result of glare and loss of contrast.

The cataract appears black against the red reflex when the eye is examined with a direct ophthalmoscope (see p. 29). Slit lamp examination allows the cataract to be examined in detail and the exact site of the opacity can be identified. Age-related cataract is commonly nuclear, cortical or subcapsular in location (Fig. 8.1). Steroid-induced cataract is commonly posterior subcapsular. Other features to suggest an ocular cause for the cataract may be found, for example pigment deposition on the lens suggesting previous inflammation or damage to the iris suggesting previous ocular trauma (Fig. 8.2).

INVESTIGATION

This is seldom required unless a suspected systemic disease requires exclusion or the cataract appears to have occurred at an early age.

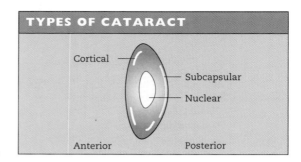

Fig. 8.1 The location of different types of cataract.

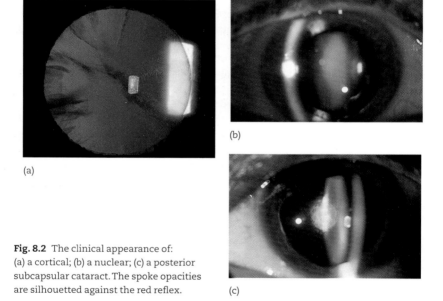

Fig. 8.2 The clinical appearance of:
(a) a cortical; (b) a nuclear; (c) a posterior
subcapsular cataract. The spoke opacities
are silhouetted against the red reflex.

TREATMENT

Although much effort has been directed towards slowing progression or to the prevention of cataract, management remains surgical. There is no need to wait for the cataract to 'ripen.' The test is whether or not the cataract produces sufficient visual symptoms to reduce the quality of life. Patients may have difficulty in recognizing faces, reading or achieving the driving standard. Some patients may be greatly troubled by glare. Patients are given some idea of their visual prognosis and must also be informed of any coexisting eye disease which may influence the outcome of cataract surgery.

Cataract surgery (Fig. 8.3)

The operation involves removal of most of the lens and its replacement optically by a plastic implant. It is increasingly performed under local rather than general anaesthesia. Local anaesthetic is infiltrated around the globe and the lids. If social circumstances allow, the patient can attend as a day case, without admission to hospital.

The operation can be performed:

• Through an extended incision at the periphery of the cornea or anterior sclera followed by *extra-capsular cataract extraction (ECCE)*.

• By liquification of the lens using an ultrasound probe introduced through a smaller incision in the cornea or anterior sclera (*phacoemulsification*).

The power of the *intraocular lens implant* to be used in the operation is calculated beforehand by measuring the length of the eye ultrasonically and the curvature of the cornea (and thus optical power) optically. The power of the lens is generally calculated so that the patient will not need glasses for distance vision. The choice of lens will also be influenced by the refraction of the fellow eye and whether it too has a cataract which may require operation. It is important that the patient is not left with a significant difference in the refractive state of the two eyes.

Postoperatively the patient is given a short course of steroid and antibiotic drops. New glasses can be prescribed after a few weeks, once the incision has healed. Since the patient cannot accomodate they will need glasses for close work even if they are not needed for distance.

Complications of cataract surgery

1 Vitreous loss. If the posterior capsule is damaged during the operation the vitreous gel may come forward into the anterior chamber where it represents a risk of glaucoma or traction on the retina. It requires removal with an instrument which aspirates and excises the gel (*vitrectomy*). In these cicumstances it may not be possible to place an intraocular lens in the eye immediately.

2 Iris prolapse. The iris may protrude through the surgical incision in the immediate postoperative period. It appears as a dark area at the incision site. The pupil is distorted. This requires prompt surgical repair.

3 Endophthalmitis. A serious but rare (less than 0.3%) infective complication of cataract extraction. Patients present with:

    (a) a painful red eye;

    (b) reduced visual acuity, usually within a few days of surgery;

    (c) a collection of white cells in the anterior chamber (hypopyon).

The patient requires urgent ophthalmic assessment, sampling of aqueous

CATARACT EXTRACTION

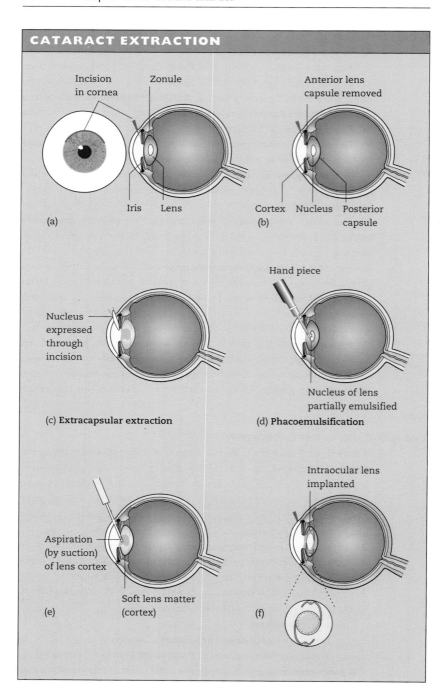

(a)

Incision in cornea
Zonule
Iris   Lens

(b)

Anterior lens capsule removed
Cortex   Nucleus   Posterior capsule

(c) **Extracapsular extraction**

Nucleus expressed through incision

(d) **Phacoemulsification**

Hand piece
Nucleus of lens partially emulsified

(e)

Aspiration (by suction) of lens cortex
Soft lens matter (cortex)

(f)

Intraocular lens implanted

and vitreous for microbiological analysis and treatment with intravitreal, topical and systemic antibiotics.

4 Postoperative astigmatism. It may be necessary to remove the corneal sutures in order to reduce corneal astigmatism. This is done prior to measuring the patient for new glasses but after the wound has healed and steroid drops have been stopped. Excessive corneal curvature can be induced in the line of the suture if it is tight. Removal usually solves this problem and is easily accomplished in the clinic under local anaesthetic with the patient sitting at the slit lamp. Loose sutures must be removed to prevent infection but it may be necessary to resuture the incision if healing is imperfect.

5 Cystoid macular oedema. The macula may become oedematous following surgery, particularly if this has been accompanied by loss of vitreous. It may settle with time but can produce a severe reduction in acuity.

6 Retinal detachment. Modern techniques of cataract extraction are associated with a low rate of this complication. It is increased if there has been vitreous loss. The symptoms, signs and management are described on p. 120.

7 Opacification of the posterior capsule (Fig. 8.4). In approximately 20% of patients clarity of the posterior capsule decreases in the months following surgery when residual epithelial cells migrate across its surface. Vision becomes blurred and there may be problems wth glare. A small hole can be made in the capsule with a laser (*neodymium yttrium (YAG) laser*) as an outpatient procedure. There is a small risk of cystoid macular oedema or retinal detachment following YAG capsulotomy.

8 If the fine nylon sutures are not removed after surgery they may break in the following months or years causing irritation or infection. Symptoms are cured by removal.

Fig. 8.3 (*Opposite.*) Stages in the removal of a cataract and the placement of an intraocular lens: (a) An incision is made in the cornea or anterior sclera. (b) The anterior capsule of the lens is removed. (c) The hard nucleus of the lens is removed through the incision, by *expression*. Pressure on the eye causes the nucleus to pass out through the incision. (d) Alternatively the nucleus can be emulsified *in situ*. The phacoemulsification probe, introduced through a small corneal or scleral incision shaves away the nucleus. (e) The remaining soft lens matter is aspirated leaving only the posterior capsule and the peripheral part of the anterior capsule. (f) An intraocular lens is implanted into the remains of the capsule. The incision is repaired with fine nylon sutures. If phacoemulsification has been used the incision in the eye is smaller and a suture may not be required.

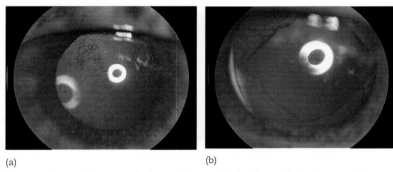

(a)   (b)

Fig. 8.4 (a) An opacified posterior capsule. (b) The result of laser capsulotomy.

Congenital cataract

The presence of congenital or infantile cataract is a threat to sight, not only because of the immediate obstruction to vision but because disturbance of the retinal image impairs visual maturation in the infant and leads to amblyopia (see p. 165). If bilateral cataract is present and has a significant effect on visual acuity this will cause amblyopia and an oscillation of the eyes (*nystagmus*). Both cataractous lenses require urgent surgery and the fitting of contact lenses to correct the aphakia. The management of contact lenses requires considerable input and motivation from the parents of the child.

The treatment of uniocular congenital cataract remains controversial. Unfortunately the results of surgery are disappointing and vision may improve little because amblyopia develops despite adequate optical correction with a contact lens. Treatment to maximize the chances of success must be performed within the first few weeks of life and accompanied by a coordinated patching routine to the fellow eye.

CHANGE IN LENS SHAPE

Abnormal lens shape is very unusual. The curvature of the anterior part of the lens may be increased centrally (*anterior lenticonus*) in Alport's syndrome, a recessively inherited condition of deafness and nephropathy. An abnormally small lens may be associated with short stature and other skeletal abnormalities.

CHANGE IN LENS POSITION (ECTOPIA LENTIS)

Weakness of the zonule causes lens displacement. The lens takes up a more rounded form and the eye becomes more myopic. This may be seen in:

- Trauma.
- Inborn errors of metabolism (e.g. Homocystinuria, a recessive disorder with mental defect and skeletal features. The lens is usually displaced downwards).
- Certain syndromes (e.g. Marfan's syndrome, a dominant disorder with skeletal and cardiac abnormalities and a risk of dissecting aortic aneurysm. The lens is usually displaced upwards). There is a defect in the zonular protein due to a mutation in the fibrillin gene.

The irregular myopia can be corrected optically although sometimes an aphakic correction may be required if the lens is substantially displaced from the visual axis. Surgical removal may be indicated, particularly if the displaced lens has caused a secondary glaucoma but surgery may result in further complications.

KEY POINTS

- In adult cataract, extraction is indicated if the reduction in vision is interfering with the patient's quality of life.
- An infant with a family history of congenital cataract or a suspected cataract must be seen by an ophthalmologist as a matter of urgency.

Box 8.3 Key points in disease of the crystalline lens.

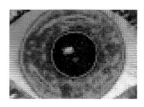

Uveitis

INTRODUCTION

Inflammation of the uveal tract, (the iris, ciliary body and choroid) has many causes and is termed *uveitis* (Fig. 9.1). It is usual for structures adjacent to the inflamed uveal tissue to become involved in the inflammatory process. It may be classified anatomically:

• Inflammation of the iris, accompanied by increased vascular permeability, is termed *iritis* or *anterior uveitis* (Fig. 9.2). White cells circulating in the aqueous humour of the anterior chamber can be seen with a slit lamp. Protein which also leaks from the blood vessels is picked out by its light scattering properties in the beam of the slit lamp as a '*flare*'.

• An inflammation of the pars plana (posterior ciliary body) is termed *cyclitis* or *intermediate uveitis*.

• Inflammation of the posterior segment (*posterior uveitis*) results in inflammatory cells in the vitreous gel. There may also be an associated choroidal or retinal inflammation (*choroiditis* and *retinitis* respectively). A *panuveitis* is present when anterior and posterior uveitis occur together.

EPIDEMIOLOGY

The incidence of uveitis is about 15 per 100 000 people. About 75% of these are anterior uveitis.

About 50% of patients with uveitis have an associated systemic disease.

HISTORY

The patient may complain of:
- ocular pain (less frequent with posterior uveitis or choroiditis);
- photophobia;
- blurring of vision;
- redness of the eye.

Posterior uveitis may not be painful.

The patient must be questioned about other relevant symptoms that may help determine whether or not there is an associated systemic disease.

- Respiratory symptoms such as shortness of breath, cough, and the nature of any sputum produced (associated sarcoidosis or tuberculosis).

- Skin problems. Erythema nodosum (painful raised red lesions on the arms and legs) may be present in granulomatous diseases such as sarcoidosis and Behçet's disease. Patients with Behçet's may also have thrombophlebitis, dermatographia and oral and genital ulceration. Psoriasis (in association with arthritis) may be accompanied by uveitis.

- Joint disease. Ankylosing spondylitis with backpain is associated with acute anterior uveitis. In children juvenile chronic arthritis may be associated with uveitis. Reiter's disease (classically urethritis, conjunctivitis and a seronegative arthritis) may also be associated with anterior uveitis.

- Bowel disease. Occasionally uveitis may be associated with inflammatory bowel diseases such as ulcerative colitis, Crohn's disease and Whipple's disease.

- Infectious disease. Syphilis with its protean manifestations can cause uveitis (particularly posterior choroiditis). Herpetic disease (shingles) may also cause uveitis. Cytomegalovirus (CMV) may cause a uveitis particularly in patients with AIDS. Fungal infections and metastatic infections may also cause uveitis, usually in immunocompromised patients.

SIGNS

On examination:
- The visual acuity may be reduced.
- The eye will be inflamed in acute anterior disease, mostly around the limbus (*ciliary injection*).
- Inflammatory cells may be visible clumped together on the endothelium of the cornea particularly inferiorly (*keratitic precipitates or KPs*).
- Slit lamp examination will reveal aqueous cells and flare. If the inflammation is severe there may be sufficient white cells to collect as a mass inferiorly (*hypopyon*).
- The vessels on the iris may be dilated.
- The iris may adhere to the lens (*posterior synechiae or PS*).

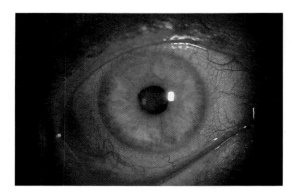

Fig. 9.1 External ocular appearance in a patient with uveitis, note the inflammatory response at the limbus.

- The intraocular pressure may be elevated.
- There may be cells in the vitreous.
- There may be retinal or choroidal foci of inflammation.
- Macular oedema may be present (see p. 117).

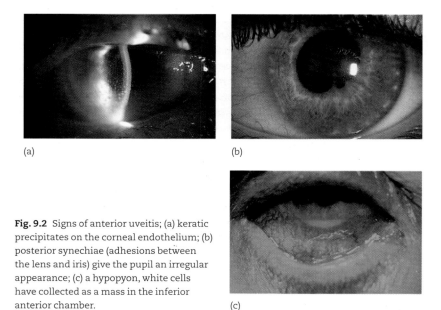

(a)

(b)

Fig. 9.2 Signs of anterior uveitis; (a) keratic precipitates on the corneal endothelium; (b) posterior synechiae (adhesions between the lens and iris) give the pupil an irregular appearance; (c) a hypopyon, white cells have collected as a mass in the inferior anterior chamber.

(c)

INVESTIGATIONS

These are aimed at determining a systemic association and are directed in part by the type of uveitis present. An anterior uveitis is more likely to be associated with ankylosing spondylitis and HLA-typing may help confirm the diagnosis (see p. 92). The presence of large KPs and possibly nodules on the iris may suggest sarcoidosis; a chest radiograph, serum calcium and serum angiotensin converting enzyme level would be appropriate. In toxoplasmic retinochoroiditis the focus of inflammation often occurs at the margin of an old inflammatory choroidal scar. A posterior uveitis may have an infectious or systemic inflammatory cause. Some diseases such as CMV virus infections in HIV positive patients have a characteristic appearance and with an appropriate history may require no further diagnostic tests. Associated symptoms may also help point towards a systemic disease (e.g. fever, diarrhoea, weight loss). Not all cases of anterior uveitis require investigation at first presentation unless associated systemic symptoms are present.

TREATMENT

This is aimed at:

- relieving pain and inflammation in the eye;
- preventing damage to ocular structures;
- preventing visual loss due to retinal or optic nerve damage.

In anterior uveitis, dilating the pupil prevents the formation of posterior synechiae by separating it from the anterior lens capsule. Synechiae otherwise interfere with normal dilatation of the pupil. Dilation is achieved with homatropine, cyclopentolate or atropine drops. Atropine drops have a prolonged action. An attempt to break any synechiae that have formed should be made with initial intensive cyclopentolate, phenylephrine and tropicamide drops. A subconjunctival injection of mydriatics may help to break resistant synechiae.

In posterior uveitis/retinitis visual loss may occur either from destructive processes caused by the retinitis itself (e.g. in toxoplasma or CMV) or from fluid accumulation in the layers of the macula (macular oedema). This may require specific antiviral or antibiotic medication or systemic steroid therapy. Some rare but severe forms of uveitis, e.g. that associated with Behçet's disease may require treatment with other systemic immunosuppresive drugs such as azathoprine or cyclosporin. Long-term treatment may be necessary.

SPECIFIC CONDITIONS ASSOCIATED WITH UVEITIS

There are a large number of systemic diseases associated with uveitis. A few of the more common ones are outlined in Table 9.1.

CAUSES OF UVEITIS

Infectious	Associated with systemic disease	Ocular disease
Toxoplasmosis	Ankylosing spondylosis	Advanced cataract
Postoperative infection	Sarcoidosis	Sympathetic ophthalmitis
Fungal	Reiter's disease	Retinal detachment
CMV	Behçet's disease	Angle closure glaucoma
Herpetic	Psoriatic arthritis	Intraocular tumours
Tuberculosis	Juvenile chronic arthritis	
Syphilis	Inflammatory bowel disease	
Metastatic infection		
Toxocara		

Table 9.1 Table showing some causes of uveitis, this is not an exclusive list.

Ankylosing spondylitis

This is a seronegative (rheumatoid factor negative) inflammatory arthritis of the spine. Genetic factors are involved in the disease. Ninety per cent of patients with uveitis have the tissue type HLA B27 although the prevalence of the disease in people in general with HLA B27 is only 1%. Approximately 20% of patients with anklyosing spondylitis will develop acute anterior uveitis. Males are affected more frequently than females (3 : 1).

HISTORY

Recurrent anterior uveitis may be the presenting feature of this condition. Close enquiry will usually reveal a history of backache, typically worse on waking and relieved by exercise. Stiffness at rest is a useful symptom which helps differentiate the condition from disease of the intervertebral discs. The peripheral joints may be affected in a minority of patients.

SIGNS

These are typical of an anterior uveitis.

INVESTIGATION

The presence of symptoms and signs in an HLA B27 positive individual is probably sufficient investigation. Sacro-iliac spinal X-rays may reveal a classical appearance of the disease.

TREATMENT

Ocular treatment is as previously outlined. The patient will benefit from a rheumatological opinion and may require intermittent anti-inflammatory treatment and physiotherapy.

PROGNOSIS

Patients may experience recurrent attacks. The outlook for vision is good if the acute attacks are treated early and vigorously.

Reiter's disease

This condition predominantly affects males, nearly all of whom are HLA B27 positive. It comprises:

- urethritis;
- arthritis (typically of the large joints);
- conjunctivitis.

Some 40% of patients develop acute anterior uveitis.

Juvenile chronic arthritis

A seronegative arthritis which presents in children, either as a systemic disease with fevers and lymphadenopathy, a pauciarticular or polyarticular arthritis. The pauciarticular form has the higher risk of chronic anterior uveitis, particularly if the patient is positive for antinuclear antibodies.

HISTORY

The anterior uveitis is chronic and usually asymptomatic. A profound visual defect may be discovered by chance if the uveitis has resulted in other ocular damage.

SIGNS

The eye is white, (unusual for iritis), but other signs of an anterior uveitis are present. Because the uveitis is chronic, cataract may occur and patients may develop glaucoma, either as a result of the uveitis or as a result of the steroid drops used to treat the condition. Approximately 70% of cases show bilateral involvement.

INVESTIGATION

Rheumatoid factor is negative but some patients have a positive antinuclear antibody.

TREATMENT

Ocular treatment is as previously outlined. Patients may be put on systemic treatment for the joint disease. It is important to screen children with juvenile arthritis regularly for uveitis as they are otherwise asymptomatic unless potentially blinding complications occur. Glaucoma can be very difficult to treat and if medical treatment fails to control pressure, it may require surgery.

Fuch's heterochromic uveitis

This is a rare chronic uveitis usually found in young adults. The cause is uncertain and there are no systemic associations.

HISTORY

The patient does not usually present with a typical history of iritis. Blurred vision and floaters may be the initial complaint.

SIGNS

A mild anterior uveitis is present but without signs of conjunctival inflammation and there are no posterior synechiae. There are KPs distributed diffusely over the cornea. The iris is heterochromic due to loss of some of the the pigment epithelial cells. The vitreous may be inflamed and condensations (the cause of the floaters) may be present. About 70% of patients develop cataract. Glaucoma occurs to a lesser extent.

TREATMENT

Steroids are not effective in controlling the inflammation and are thus not prescribed. The patients usually respond well to cataract surgery when it is required. The glaucoma is treated conventionally.

Toxoplasmosis (Fig. 9.3)

HISTORY

The infection may be congenital or acquired. Most ocular toxoplasmosis (50–75%) is thought to be congenital but the resulting retinochoroiditis heals in infancy and a reactivated lesion presents in adult life. The patient may complain of hazy vision, floaters, and the eye may be red and painful.

SIGNS

The retina is the principal structure involved with secondary inflammation occuring in the choroid. An active lesion is often located at the posterior pole, appearing as a creamy focus of inflammatory cells at the margin of an old chorioretinal scar (such scars are usually atrophic, with a pigmented

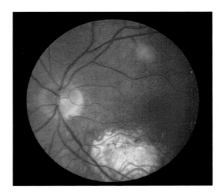

Fig. 9.3 The appearance of an inactive Toxoplasma retinitis.

edge). Inflammatory cells cause a vitreous haze and the anterior chamber may also show evidence of inflammation.

INVESTIGATION

The clinical appearance is usually diagnostic but a positive toxoplasma antibody test is suggestive. However, a high percentage of the population have positive IgG titres due to prior infection.

TREATMENT

The reactivated lesions will subside but treatment is required if the macula or optic nerve is threatened or if the inflammatory response is very severe. Systemic steroids are administered with an antiprotozoal such as clindamycin. Care must be taken with the treatment as pseudomembranous colitis may result from clindamycin treatment. Patients must be warned that if diarrhoea develops they should seek medical help immediately.

Acquired immunodeficiency syndrome (AIDS) and CMV retinitis (Fig. 9.4)

Ocular disease is a common manifestation of the acquired immunodeficiency syndrome. Patients develop a variety of ocular conditions:
- microvascular occlusion causing retinal haemorrhages and cotton wool spots (infarcted areas of the nerve fibre layer of the retina);
- corneal endothelial deposits;
- neoplasms of the eye and orbit;
- neuro-ophthalmic disorders including oculomotor palsies;

- opportunistic infections of which the most common is CMV retinitis, (it may develop in more than one-third of AIDS patients). Toxoplasmosis, Herpes simplex and Herpes zoster are amongst other infections that may be seen.

HISTORY

The patient may complain of blurred vision or floaters. A diagnosis of HIV disease has usually already been made, often other AIDS defining features have occured.

SIGNS

CMV retinopathy comprises a whitish area of retina, associated with haemorrhage, which has been likened in appearance to 'cottage cheese'. The lesions may threaten the macula or the optic disc. There is usually an associated sparse inflammation of the vitreous.

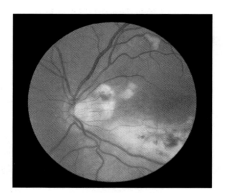

Fig. 9.4 The retinal appearance in a patient with AIDS and CMV retinitis. (Note the cotton wool spot at one o'clock.)

TREATMENT

Chronic therapy with Ganciclovir and/or Foscarnet given parenterally are the current mainstay of therapy. Ganciclovir is also available orally. Systems of depot delivery into the vitreous are being actively researched for local ocular CMV retinitis.

PROGNOSIS

Prolonged treatment is required to prevent recurrence.

SYMPATHETIC OPHTHALMITIS

A penetrating or surgical injury to one eye involving the retina may rarely excite a peculiar form of uveitis which involves not only the injured eye but also the fellow eye. This is termed sympathetic ophthalmitis (or ophthalmia). The uveitis may be so severe that in the worst cases sight may be lost from both eyes. Fortunately systemic steroids have greatly improved the chances of conserving vision. Sympathetic ophthalmitis usually develops within 3 months of the injury or last ocular operation but may occur at any time. The cause appears due to an immune response against retinal antigens at the time of injury. It can be prevented by enucleation (removal) of the traumatized eye shortly (within a week or so) after the injury if the prospects for visual potential in that eye are very poor and there is major disorganization.

SYMPTOMS

The patient may complain of pain and decreased vision in the seeing eye.

SIGNS

The iris appears swollen and yellow-white spots may be seen on the retina. There is a panuveitis.

TREATMENT

High-dose systemic and topical steroids are required to reduce the inflammation and try to prevent long term visual loss. It is vital to warn patients with ocular trauma or multiple eye operations to attend an eye casualty department if they experience any problems with their normal eye.

KEY POINTS

- Angle closure glaucoma may cause an anterior uveitis and may present with similar symptoms. Look for a dilated pupil and check the intraocular pressure.
- Patients with a retinal detachment may occasionally present with an anterior uveitis. The retina should always be examined in patients with uveitis.
- Active treatment of uveitis is required to prevent long term complications.
- Children with juvenile arthritis require regular screening to exclude the presence of uveitis as it is usually asymptomatic.

Box 9.1 Key points in uveitis.

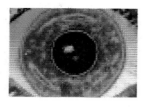

Glaucoma

INTRODUCTION

The glaucomas comprise a group of diseases in which damage to the optic nerve (optic neuropathy) is usually caused by the effects of raised ocular pressure acting at the optic nerve head. Independent ischaemia of the optic nerve head may also be important. Axon loss results in visual field defects and a loss of visual acuity if the central visual field is involved.

BASIC PHYSIOLOGY (Fig. 10.1)

The intraocular pressure level depends on the balance between production and removal of aqueous humour. Aqueous is produced by secretion and ultrafiltration from the ciliary processes into the posterior chamber. It then passes through the pupil into the anterior chamber to leave the eye predominantly via the trabecular meshwork, Schlemm's canal and the episcleral veins (*the conventional pathway*). A small proportion of the aqueous (4%) drains across the ciliary body into the supra-choroidal space and into the venous circulation across the sclera (*uveoscleral pathway*).

Two theories have been advanced for the mechanism by which an elevated intraocular pressure damages nerve fibres:
• Raised intraocular pressure causes mechanical damage to the optic nerve axons.
• Raised intraocular pressure causes ischaemia of the nerve axons by reducing bloodflow at the optic nerve head.

Probably the pathophysiology of glaucoma is multifactorial and both mechanisms are important.

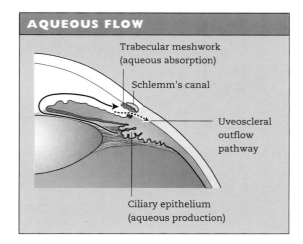

AQUEOUS FLOW

Trabecular meshwork
(aqueous absorption)

Schlemm's canal

Uveoscleral
outflow
pathway

Ciliary epithelium
(aqueous production)

Fig. 10.1 Diagram of the drainage angle showing routes taken by aqueous from production to absorption.

CLASSIFICATION

The mechanism by which absorption is reduced provides a means of classifying the glaucomas (Fig. 10.2).

CLASSIFICATION OF GLAUCOMAS

Primary glaucoma	• Chronic open angle
	• Acute and chronic closed angle
Congenital glaucoma	• Primary
	• Rubella
	• Secondary to other inherited ocular disorders (i.e. aniridia, absence of the iris).
Secondary glaucoma (causes)	• Trauma
	• Ocular surgery
	• Associated with other ocular disease (e.g. uveitis)
	• Raised episcleral venous pressure
	• Steroid induced

Box 10.1 Classification of the glaucomas.

Classification of the primary glaucomas is based on whether or not the iris is:
• clear of the trabecular meshwork (*open angle*);
• covering the meshwork (*closed angle*).

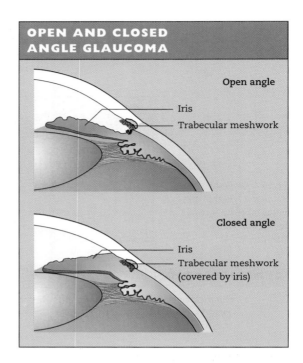

OPEN AND CLOSED ANGLE GLAUCOMA

Open angle

Iris

Trabecular meshwork

Closed angle

Iris

Trabecular meshwork (covered by iris)

Fig. 10.2 Diagram showing the difference between open and closed angle glaucoma.

PATHOGENESIS

Primary open angle glaucoma

A special contact lens (gonioscopy lens) applied to the cornea allows a view of the iridocorneal angle with the slit lamp. In open angle glaucoma the structure of the trabecular meshwork appears normal but offers an increased resistance to the outflow of aqueous which results in an elevated ocular pressure. The causes of outflow obstruction include:

• thickening of the trabecular lamellae which reduces pore size;
• reduction in the number of lining trabecular cells;
• increased extracellular material in the trabecular meshwork.

A form of glaucoma also exists in which glaucomatous field loss and cupping of the optic disc occurs although the intraocular pressure is not raised (*normal or low tension glaucoma*). It is thought that the optic nerve head in these patients is unusually susceptible to the intraocular pressure or has intrinsically reduced blood flow (Fig. 10.3).

Conversely, intraocular pressure may be raised without evidence of visual damage or pathological optic disc cupping (*ocular hypertension*). These subjects may represent the extreme end of the normal range of intraocular pressure, however, a small proportion will subsequently develop glaucoma.

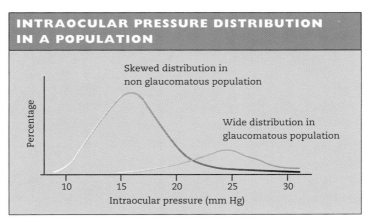

Fig. 10.3 The distribution of intraocular pressure in a normal and glaucomatous population.

Closed angle glaucoma

The condition occurs in small eyes (i.e. often hypermetropic) with shallow anterior chambers. In the normal eye the point of contact between the pupil margin and the lens offers a resistance to aqueous entry into the anterior chamber (relative pupil block). In angle closure glaucoma, sometimes in response to pupil dilation, this resistance is increased and the pressure gradient created bows the iris forward and closes the drainage angle. Aqueous can no longer drain through the trabecular meshwork and ocular pressure rises, usually abruptly.

Secondary glaucoma

Intraocular pressure usually rises in secondary glaucoma due to blockage of the trabecular meshwork. The trabecular meshwork may be blocked by:
- Blood (*hyphaema*), following blunt trauma.
- Inflammatory cells (*uveitis*).
- Pigment from the iris (*pigment dispersion syndrome*).
- Deposition of material produced by the epithelium of the lens, iris and ciliary body in the trabecular meshwork (*pseudoexfoliative glaucoma*).

- Drugs increasing the resistance of the meshwork (*steroid-induced glaucoma*).

Secondary glaucoma may also result from blunt trauma to the eye damaging the angle (*angle recession*).

Angle closure may also account for some cases of secondary glaucoma:

- Abnormal iris blood vessels may obstruct the angle and cause the iris to adhere to the peripheral cornea, closing the angle (*rubeosis iridis*). This may accompany proliferative diabetic retinopathy or central retinal vein occlusion due to the forward diffusion of vasoproliferative factors from the ischaemic retina (Fig. 10.4).

- A large choroidal melanoma may push the iris forward approximating it to the peripheral cornea causing an acute attack of angle closure glaucoma.

- A cataract may swell, pushing the iris forward and closing the drainage angle.

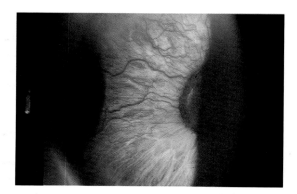

Fig. 10.4 The appearance of the rubeotic iris, note the irregular pattern of the new blood vessels on the surface.

Raised episcleral venous pressure is an unusual cause of glaucoma but may be seen in *caroticocavernous sinus fistula* where a connection between the carotid artery or its meningeal branches and the cavernous sinus, causes a marked elevation in orbital venous pressure. It is also thought to be the cause of the raised intraocular pressure in patients with the *Sturge–Weber Syndrome*.

The cause of congenital glaucoma remains uncertain. The iridocorneal angle may be developmentally abnormal, and covered with a membrane.

Chronic open angle glaucoma

EPIDEMIOLOGY

Chronic open angle glaucoma affects 1 in 200 of the population over the age of 40, affecting males and females equally. The prevalence increases with age to nearly 10% in the over 80 population. There may be a family history, although the exact mode of inheritance is not clear. Subjects with a first degree relative with glaucoma are more likely to develop the disease than those with no family history.

HISTORY

The symptoms of glaucoma depend on the rate at which intraocular pressure rises. Chronic open angle glaucoma is associated with a slow rise in pressure and is symptomless unless the patient becomes aware of a severe visual deficit. Many patients are diagnosed when the signs of glaucoma are detected by their optometrist.

EXAMINATION   (Fig. 10.5)

Assessment of a glaucoma suspect requires a full slit lamp examination:

- To measure ocular pressure with a tonometer. The normal pressure is 15.5 mmHg. The upper limit is defined as 2 standard deviations above the mean (21 mmHg). In chronic open angle glaucoma the pressure is typically in the 22–40 mmHg (in angle closure glaucoma it rises above 60 mmHg).
- To examine the iridocorneal angle with the gonioscopy lens to confirm that an open angle is present.
- To examine the optic disc and determine whether it is pathologically cupped. Cupping is a normal feature of the optic disc (Fig. 10.5(a)). The disc is assessed by estimating the vertical ratio of the cup to the disc as a whole (the cup to disc ratio) (Fig. 10.5). In the normal eye the cup disc ratio is usually no greater than 0.4. There is a considerable range (0–0.8) and the size of the cup is related to the size of the disc. In chronic glaucoma, axons entering the optic nervehead die. The central cup expands and the rim of nerve fibres (neuroretinal rim) becomes thinner. The nervehead becomes atrophic. The cup to disc ratio in the vertical is greater than 0.4 and the cup deepens. If the cup is deep but the cup to disc ratio is lower than 0.4, then chronic glaucoma is unlikely. Notching of the rim may also be a sign of glaucomatous damage.
- To exclude a secondary cause for the glaucoma.

Field testing (perimetry see pp. 21–23) is used to establish the presence of islands of field loss (scotomata) and to follow patients to determine

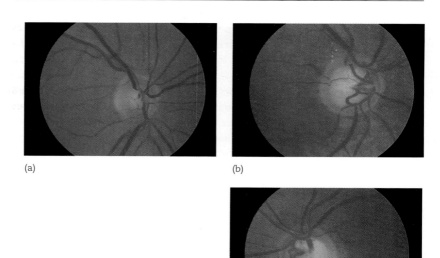

(a)   (b)

Fig. 10.5 Comparison of (a) a normal optic disc; (b) a glaucomatous optic disc; (c) a disc haemorrhage is a feature of patients with low tension glaucoma.

(c)

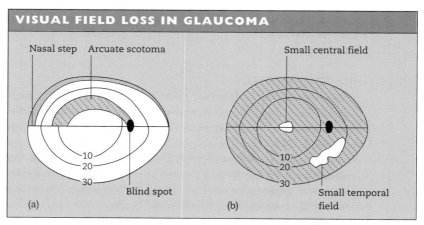

VISUAL FIELD LOSS IN GLAUCOMA

Nasal step   Arcuate scotoma   Small central field

10
20
30

Blind spot   Small temporal
(a)   (b)   field

Fig. 10.6 The characteristic pattern of visual field loss in chronic open angle glaucoma: (a) an upper arcuate scotoma, reflecting damage to a cohort of nerve fibres entering the lower pole of the disc (remember—the optics of the eye determine that damage to the lower retina creates an upper field defect; (b) the field loss has progressed, a small central island is left (tunnel vision), sometimes this may be associated with a sparing of an island of vision in the temporal field.

whether visual damage is progressive (Fig. 10.6). A proportion of nerve fibres may, however, be damaged before field loss becomes apparent. This has stimulated the search for more sensitive means of assessing visual function with different forms of perimetry (a blue target on a yellow background instead of a *white* target on a *white* background), and testing sensitivity to motion in the peripheral visual field. As yet no better test has been developed for clinical use.

SYMPTOMS AND SIGNS	
Chronic open angle glaucoma	• symptomless
	• raised intraocular pressure
	• visual field defect
	• cupped optic disc

Box 10.2 Symptoms and signs of chronic open angle glaucoma.

TREATMENT

Treatment is aimed at reducing intraocular pressure. The level to which the pressure must be lowered varies from patient to patient, and is that which minimises further glaucomatous visual loss. This requires careful monitoring in the outpatient clinic. Three modalities of treatment are available:

1 medical treatment;
2 laser treatment;
3 surgical treatment.

MEDICAL TREATMENT

Topical drugs commonly used in the treatment of glaucoma are listed in Table 10.1. In chronic open angle glaucoma topical adrenergic beta-blockers are the usual first line treatment. These act by reducing aqueous production. Selective agents, which may have fewer systemic side effects, are available but must still be used with caution in those with respiratory disease, particularly asthma, which may be exacerbated even by the small amount of beta-blocker absorbed systemically. If intraocular pressure remains elevated the choice lies between:

• adding additional medical treatment;
• laser treatment;
• surgical drainage procedures.

LASER TRABECULOPLASTY

This involves placing a series of laser burns (50 µm wide) in the trabecular meshwork, to improve aqueous outflow. Whilst effective initially, the

TREATMENT OF GLAUCOMA

Topical Agents	Action	Side-effects
Beta-blockers (Timolol)	Decrease secretion	Exacerbate asthma and chronic airway disease. Hypotension, bradycardia.
Parasympathomimetic (pilocarpine) central	Increase outflow	Visual blurring in young patients and those with cataracts. Initially, headache due to ciliary spasm.
Sympathomimetic (adrenaline)	Increase outflow	Redness of the eye. Headache.
Carbonic anhydrase inhibitor (dorzolamide)	Decrease secretion	Stinging. Unpleasant taste. Headache.
Systemic Agents		
Carbonic anhydrase inhibitors (acetazolamide)	Decrease secretion	Tingling in limbs. Depression, sleepiness. Renal stones. Stevens–Johnson Syndrome

Table 10.1 Examples and mode of action of drugs used in the treatment of glaucoma. Side effects occur with variable frequency.

intraocular pressure may slowly increase. In the UK there is an increasing tendency to proceed to early drainage surgery.

SURGICAL TREATMENT

Drainage surgery (*trabeculectomy*) relies on the creation of a fistula between the anterior chamber and the subconjunctival space (Fig. 10.7). The operation is usually effective in substantially reducing intraocular pressure. It is performed increasingly early in the treatment of glaucoma.

Complications of surgery include:
- shallowing of the anterior chamber in the immediate post-operative period risking damage to the lens and cornea;
- intraocular infection;
- possibly accelerated cataract development.

Recent evidence suggests that some topical medications, particularly sympathomimetic agents, may increase conjunctival scarring and reduce the chances of a successful operation when the new drainage channel becomes scarred and non-functional.

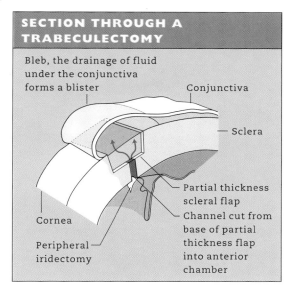

(a)

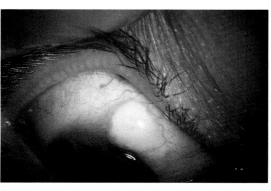

(b)

Fig. 10.7 (a) Diagram showing a section through a trabeculectomy. An incision is made in the conjunctiva, which is dissected and reflected to expose bare sclera. A partial thickness scleral flap is then fashioned. Just anterior to the scleral spur a small opening (termed a *sclerostomy*) is made into the anterior chamber to create a low resistance drain for aqueous. The iris is excised in the region of the sclerostomy (*iridectomy*) to prevent it moving forward and blocking the opening. The partial thickness flap is loosely sutured back into place. The conjunctiva is tightly sutured. Aqueous can now leak through the sclerostomy, around and through the scleral flap and underneath the conjunctiva where it forms a bleb. (b) The appearance of a trabeculectomy bleb.

Normal tension glaucoma, considered to lie at one end of the spectrum of chronic open angle glaucoma, can be particularly difficult to treat. Some patients appear to have non-progressive visual field defects and require no treatment. In those with progressive field loss lowering intraocular pressure may be beneficial.

Each form of treatment has its complications and therapy must be aimed at minimising these whilst maximising effectiveness.

Primary angle closure glaucoma (Fig. 10.8)

EPIDEMIOLOGY

Primary angle closure glaucoma affects 1 in 1000 subjects over 40 years old, with females more commonly affected than males. Patients with angle closure glaucoma are likely to be long-sighted because the long-sighted eye is small and the anterior chamber structures more crowded.

HISTORY

In acute angle closure glaucoma, there is an abrupt increase in pressure and the eye becomes very painful and photophobic. There is watering of the eye and loss of vision. The patient may be systemically unwell with nausea and abdominal pain, symptoms which may take them to a general casualty department.

Intermittent primary angle closure glaucoma occurs when an acute attack spontaneously resolves. The patient may complain of pain, blurring of vision and seeing haloes around lights.

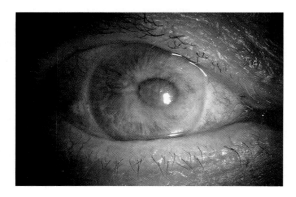

Fig. 10.8 The appearance of the eye in angle closure glaucoma. Note the cloudy cornea and dilated pupil.

EXAMINATION

On examination visual acuity is reduced, the eye red, the cornea cloudy and the pupil oval, fixed and dilated.

TREATMENT

The acute and dramatic rise in pressure seen in angle closure glaucoma must be urgently countered to prevent permanent damage to the vision. Acetazolamide is administered intravenously and subsequently orally together with topical pilocarpine and beta-blockers. Pilocarpine constricts the pupil and draws the peripheral iris out of the angle; the acetazolamide and beta blocker reduce aqueous secretion and the pressure across the iris. These measures usually break the attack and lower intraocular pressure. Subsequent management requires that a small hole (*iridotomy or iridectomy*) is made in the peripheral iris to prevent subsequent attacks, to provide an alternative pathway to the pupil, for fluid to flow from the posterior to the anterior chamber reducing the pressure gradient across the iris. This can be done with a YAG laser or surgically. If the pressure has been raised for some days the iris becomes adherent to the peripheral cornea (*peripheral anterior synechiae* or *PAS*). The iridocorneal angle is damaged and additional medical or surgical measures may be required to lower the ocular pressure.

Secondary glaucoma

Secondary glaucomas are much rarer than the primary glaucomas. The symptoms and signs depend on the rate at which intraocular pressure rises; most are again symptomless. Treatment broadly follows the lines of the primary disease. In secondary glaucoma it is important to treat any underlying cause, e.g. uveitis, which may be responsible for the glaucoma.

In particularly difficult cases it may be necessary to selectively ablate the ciliary processes in order to reduce aqueous production. This is done by application of a laser or cryoprobe to the sclera overlying the processes. Endoscopic techniques are also under development.

Congenital glaucoma

This covers a diverse range of disease. It may present at birth or within the first year. Symptoms and signs include:
*   excessive tearing;
*   an increased corneal diameter (*buphthalmos*);
*   a cloudy cornea due to epithelial oedema;

- splits in Descemet's membrane.

Congenital glaucoma is usually treated surgically. An incision is made into the trabecular meshwork (*goniotomy*) to increase aqueous drainage or a direct passage between Schlemm's canal and the anterior chamber is created (*trabeculotomy*).

Prognosis of the glaucomas

The goal of treatment in glaucoma is to stop or reduce the rate of visual damage. It may be that control of intraocular pressure alone is not the only factor that needs to be addressed in the management of glaucoma although it is currently the mainstay of treatment. Some patients will continue to develop visual loss despite a large decrease in intraocular pressure. Nonetheless vigorous lowering of intraocular pressure even when it does not prevent continued visual loss appears to significantly reduce the rate of progression.

If intraocular pressure remains controlled following acute treatment of angle closure glaucoma progressive visual damage is unlikely. The same applies to the secondary glaucomas if treatment of the underlying cause results in a reduction of intraocular pressure into the normal range.

KEY POINTS

- Glaucoma is an optic neuropathy caused by an elevation of intraocular pressure.
- Primary glaucoma is classified according to whether the trabecular meshwork is obstructed by the peripheral iris (angle closure) or not (open angle glaucoma).
- Treatment of glaucoma relies on lowering ocular pressure to reduce or prevent further visual damage.
- Ocular pressure can be reduced with topical and systemic medications, laser treatment and surgery.
- Beware patients who are acutely debilitated with a red eye, they may have acute angle closure glaucoma.

Box 10.3 Glaucoma key points.

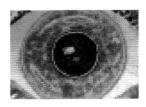

Retina and choroid

INTRODUCTION

The retina is subject to an enormous range of disease, both inherited and acquired. Some are common, with significant socio-economic importance (age related macular degeneration) while others are much rarer (for example some of the macular dystrophies). The impact on the individual may be profound in either case. Diseases of the macula, particularly if bilateral, result in a profound reduction in visual acuity. Despite the enormous range of disease the symptoms are relatively constant. These will be described first. In this chapter both hereditary and acquired disease of the vitreous, neuroretina, retinal pigment epithelium and choroid will be described. In the chapter which follows the effects of disorders of the retinal circulation will be explored.

SYMPTOMS OF RETINAL DISEASE

Macular dysfunction

The central part of the macula (the fovea) is responsible for fine resolu-

tion. Disorders of this relatively small part of the retina cause significant visual impairment. The patient may complain of:
• Blurred central vision.
• Distorted vision (*metamorphopsia*) caused by a disturbance in the arrangement of the photoreceptors such as that which occurs in macular oedema. A reduction (*micropsia*) or enlargement (*macropsia*) of object size may also occur if the photoreceptors become compressed together or stretched apart.
• The patient may notice areas of loss of the central visual field (*scotomata*) if part of the photoreceptor layer becomes covered, e.g. by blood, or if the photoreceptors are destroyed.

Peripheral retinal dysfunction

The patient complains of:
• Loss of visual field (usually detected clinically when a significant amount of the peripheral retina is damaged). Small areas of damage, e.g. small haemorrhages, do not produce clinically detectable defects. The field loss may be absolute for example in a branch retinal artery occlusion or relative (that is brighter or larger objects are visible) as in a retinal detachment.
• Some diseases affecting the retina may predominantly affect one type of photoreceptor; in retinitis pigmentosa the rods are principally affected so that night vision is reduced (night blindness).

ACQUIRED MACULAR DISEASE

Acquired disease at the macula may destroy part or all of the retina or retinal pigment epithelial layers (e.g. age related macular degeneration or a macular hole). In a number of conditions this damage is dramatically magnified by the growth of new vessels from the choroid through Bruch's membrane and the retinal pigment epithelium to cause haemorrhage or exudation of fluid into the subretinal space and subsequent scarring of the retina. The retina ceases to function if it is detached from the retinal pigment epithelium so that these changes cause marked disruption of macular function even before direct retinal damage occurs.

Fluid may also accumulate within the layers of the retina at the macula (*cystoid macular oedema*) if the normal tight junctions of the retinal capillaries that form the blood–retinal barrier break down. This may occur following intraocular surgery, such as cataract surgery. The retina and subretinal layers may also become separated by diffusion of fluid from the choriocapillaris through an abnormal region of the retinal pigment epithelium. This represents a breakdown of the deep part of the blood-retina barrier between the choroid and the retina and is termed central-serous retinopathy. It may occur unilaterally, as a potentially reversible disorder in young men.

Age related macular degeneration (Fig. 11.1)

Age related macular degeneration (ARMD) is the commonest cause of irreversible visual loss in the developed world.

PATHOGENESIS

Lipid products are found in Bruch's membrane. They are thought to arise from the outer segments of the photoreceptors due to failure of the retinal pigment epithelium (RPE) to remove this material. Deposits form which can be seen with the ophthalmoscope as discrete sub-retinal yellow lesions called drusen. The RPE and the photoreceptors also show degen-

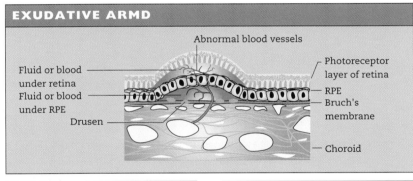

EXUDATIVE ARMD

Abnormal blood vessels

Fluid or blood under retina

Fluid or blood under RPE

Drusen

Photoreceptor layer of retina

RPE

Bruch's membrane

Choroid

(a)

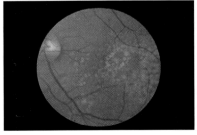

(b)

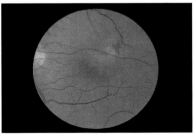

(c)

Fig. 11.1 (a) The pathogenesis of exudative age related macular degeneration (RPE, retinal pigment epithelium). Pictures of: (b) dry ARMD, note the discrete scattered yellowish sub-retinal drusen; (c) wet ARMD, note the small haemorrhage associated with the sub-retinal membrane.

erative changes. This is the dry or non-exudative form of age related macular degeneration (ARMD). In the less common exudative (wet) form new vessels from the choroid grow through Bruch's membrane and the retinal pigment epithelial layer into the sub-retinal space where they form a *sub-retinal neovascular membrane*. Subsequent haemorrhage into the sub-retinal space or even through the retina into the vitreous is associated with profound visual loss.

SYMPTOMS

The symptoms are those of macular dysfunction outlined above.

SIGNS

The usual foveal reflex is absent. Yellow, well-circumscribed drusen may be seen and there may be areas of hypo- and hyperpigmentation. In exudative ARMD sub-retinal, or more occasionally pre-retinal, haemorrhages may be seen. The experienced observer may detect elevation of the retina stereoscopically.

INVESTIGATION

Diagnosis is based on the appearance of the retina. In patients with a suspected exudative ARMD and with vision that is not severely affected a fluorescein angiogram may be performed to deliniate the position of the sub-retinal neovascular membrane. The position of the membrane determines whether or not the patient may benefit from laser treatment.

TREATMENT

There is no treatment for non-exudative ARMD. Vision is maximized with low vision aids including magnifiers and telescopes. The patient is assured that although central vision has been lost, the disease does not cause a loss of peripheral vision. This is vital as many patients fear that they will become totally blind.

In a small proportion of patients with exudative ARMD, where the fluorescein angiogram shows the subretinal vascular membrane to lie eccentric to the fovea, it may be possible to obliterate it with argon-laser treatment. Unfortunately even with laser treatment the condition can recur.

OTHER DEGENERATIVE CONDITIONS ASSOCIATED WITH THE FORMATION OF SUB-RETINAL NEOVASCULAR MEMBRANES

- Degenerative changes at the macula and the formation of sub-retinal neovascular membranes may also be seen in very myopic patients, this can cause loss of central vision particularly in young adulthood.

• Sub-retinal neovascular membranes may also grow through elongated cracks in Bruch's membrane called *angioid streaks*. Angioid streaks may be associated with systemic diseases, such as Paget's disease, occasionally sickle cell disease and the rare recessive disorder, pseudoxanthoma elasticum. Again there may be a profound reduction in central vision. Vision is also reduced if the crack itself passes through the fovea (Fig. 11.2).

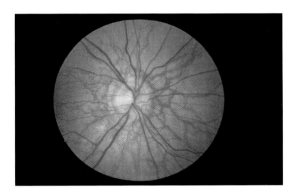

Fig. 11.2 The clinical appearance of angioid streaks.

Macular holes and membranes (Fig. 11.3)

A well-circumscribed hole may form in the macular region and destroy the fovea. It results from traction by the vitreous on the thin macular retina. Again there is a profound loss of central vision. The early stages of hole formation may be associated with distortion and mild blurring of vision.

Unlike peripheral retinal holes, macular holes are not usually associated with retinal detachments. Most are idiopathic in origin but they may be associated with blunt trauma. Much interest is being shown in the treatment of macular holes with vitreous surgery to relieve the traction on the retina. No other treatment is available.

A pre-retinal glial membrane may form over the macular region, whose contraction causes puckering of the retina and again results in blurring and distortion of vision. These symptoms may be improved by removing the membrane with microsurgical vitrectomy techniques.

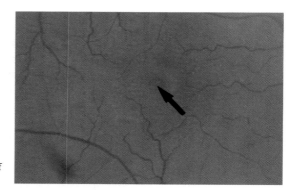

Fig. 11.3 The appearance of a macular hole.

Central-serous retinopathy (Fig. 11.4)

This localized accumulation of fluid between the retina and the RPE causes the separation of the two layers and distortion of the photoreceptor layer. It results from a localized breakdown in the normal structure of the RPE. Typically it affects young or middle-aged males. Patients complain of distortion and blurred vision. Examination reveals a dome-shaped elevation of the retina.

Treatment is not usually required as the condition is self-limiting. Occasionally in intractable cases, or those where the vision is severely affected, the argon laser can be used to seal the point of leakage identified with a fluorescein angiogram.

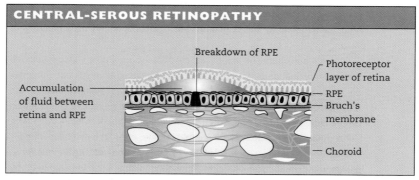

Fig. 11.4 The pattern of fluid accumulation in central-serous retinopathy.

Macular oedema (Fig. 11.5)

This accumulation of fluid within the retina itself is a further cause of distorted and blurred vision. Ophthalmoscopy reveals a loss of the normal foveal reflex and with experience a rather cystic appearance to the fovea. If the diagnosis is in doubt a confirmatory fluorescein angiogram can be performed. The fluorescein leaks out into the oedematous retina (see p. 34).

Macular oedema may be associated with numerous and diverse eye disorders including:

- intraocular surgery;
- uveitis;
- retinal vascular disease (e.g. diabetic retinopathy);
- retinitis pigmentosa.

Treatment can be difficult and is dependent on the associated eye disease. Steroids in high doses are helpful in macular oedema caused by uveitis; acetazolamide may be helpful in treating patients with retinitis pigmentosa or following intraocular surgery.

Prolonged macular oedema can cause the formation of a lamellar macular hole.

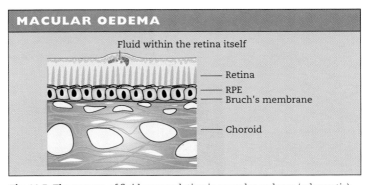

MACULAR OEDEMA

Fluid within the retina itself

Retina
RPE
Bruch's membrane

Choroid

Fig. 11.5 The pattern of fluid accumulation in macular oedema (schematic).

Toxic maculopathies (Fig. 11.6)

The accumulation of some drugs in the RPE can cause macular damage. These include the antimalarials chloroquine and hydroxychloroquine, used quite widely in the treatment of rheumatoid arthritis and other connective tissue disorders, which may cause a toxic maculopathy. Chloroquine is the more toxic. Patients on chloroquine require regular ophthalmic screening for maculopathy. The maculopathy is initially only detected by accurate assessment of macular function. At this early stage, discontinuation of the drug results in reversal. Later, a pigmentary target lesion is seen ophthalmoscopically associated with metamorphopsia and an irreversible and appreciable loss of central vision. Ocular toxicity is unlikely with a dose of less than 4 mg (chloroquine phosphate) per kg lean body-weight per day or a total cumulative dose of less than 300 g. Screening of patients on hydroxychloroquine, although still advised, is questioned by some.

Phenothiazines used in high doses for prolonged periods (in the treatment of psychoses) may cause retinal damage.

Tamoxifen, in high doses, may cause a maculopathy.

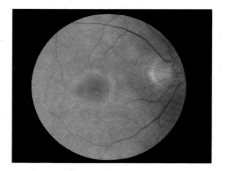

Fig. 11.6 Bull's-eye appearance in chloroquine maculopathy.

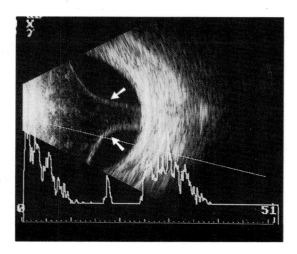

Fig. 11.7 Ultrasound picture showing a posterior vitreous detachment. Note that the vitreous is still attached at the optic disc and the ora serrata.

POSTERIOR VITREOUS DETACHMENT (Fig. 11.7)

The vitreous gel undergoes degenerative changes in patients in their 50s and 60s (earlier in myopes) causing it to detach from the retina. This produces floaters.

These are a common symptom particularly in middle aged patients. They take the form of spots or cobwebs which move when the eye moves and obscure vision only slightly. The symptom is caused by shadows cast on the retina by fragments of condensed vitreous. The symptom is most marked on bright days when the small pupil throws a sharper image on the retina. Sometimes the vitreous, which is relatively loosely attached to most of the retina detaches, a condition termed a *posterior vitreous detachment*. This gives rise to acute symptoms of:

- *Photopsia* (flashing lights). This results from traction on the retina by the detaching vitreous.
- A shower of floaters. This is common and sometimes may indicate a vitreous haemorrhage when the detaching vitreous ruptures a small blood vessel.

RETINAL DETACHMENT

PATHOGENESIS

The potential space between the neuroretina and its pigment epithelium corresponds to the cavity of the embryonic optic vesicle. The two tissues are loosely attached in the mature eye and may become separated:

- if a tear occurs in the retina, allowing liquified vitreous to gain entry to the subretinal space and causing a progressive detachment (*rhegmatogenous retinal detachment*);
- if it is pulled off by contracting fibrous tissue on the retinal surface (e.g. as in the proliferative retinopathy of diabetes mellitus (*tractional retinal detachment*);
- when, rarely, fluid accumulates in the subretinal space as a result of an exudative process, which may occur during toxaemia of pregnancy (*exudative retinal detachment*).

Tears in the retina are most commonly associated with the onset of a posterior vitreous detachment. As the gel separates from the retina the traction it exerts (*vitreous traction*) becomes more localized and thus greater. Occasionally it may be sufficient to tear the retina. An underlying peripheral weakness of the retina such as *lattice degeneration*, increases the probability of a tear forming when the vitreous pulls on the retina.

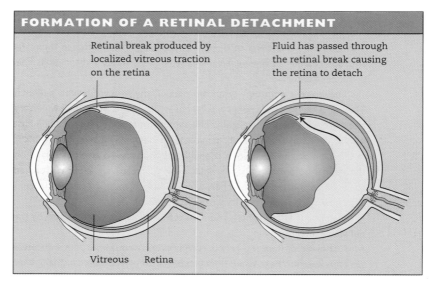

FORMATION OF A RETINAL DETACHMENT

Retinal break produced by localized vitreous traction on the retina

Fluid has passed through the retinal break causing the retina to detach

Vitreous   Retina

Fig. 11.8 The formation of a rhegmatogenous retinal detachment. (a) The detaching vitreous has torn the retina. The vitreous continues to pull on the retina surrounding the break (vitreous traction). (b) Fluid from the vitreous cavity passes through the break detaching the retina from the underlying retinal pigment epithelium.

Rhegmatogenous retinal detachment (Fig. 11.8)

EPIDEMIOLOGY

About 1 in 10 000 of the normal population will suffer a rhegmatogenous retinal detachment. The probability is increased in patients who:
- are high myopes;
- have undergone cataract surgery, particularly if this was complicated by vitreous loss;
- have experienced a detached retina in the fellow eye;
- have been subjected to recent severe eye trauma.

SYMPTOMS

Retinal detachment may be preceded by symptoms of a posterior vitreous detachment, including floaters and flashing lights. With the onset of the retinal detachment itself the patient notices the progressive development of a field defect, often described as a 'shadow' or 'curtain'. Progression may be rapid when a superior detachment is present. If the macula becomes detached there is a marked fall in visual acuity.

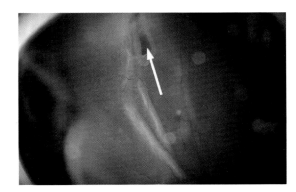

Fig. 11.9 The clinical appearance of a retinal detachment; note the retinal tear. The retina has completely detached.

SIGNS

The detached retina is visible on ophthalmoscopy as a pinkish greyish membrane which partly obscures the choroidal vascular detail. If there is a marked accumulation of fluid in the sub-retinal space (a *bullous retinal detachment*) undulating movements of the retina will be observed as the eye moves. A tear in the retina appears reddish pink because of the underlying choroidal vessels. There may be associated debris in the vitreous comprising blood (*vitreous haemorrhage*) and pigment, or the lid (*operculum*) of a retinal hole may be found floating free (Fig. 11.9).

MANAGEMENT   (Fig. 11.10)

There are two major surgical techniques for repairing a retinal detachment:

1   external (*conventional approach*);
2   internal (*vitreoretinal surgery*).

The essential principle behind both techniques is to close the causative break in the retina and to increase the strength of attachment between the surrounding retina and the retinal pigment epithelium by inducing inflammation in the region either by local freezing with a cryoprobe or with a laser. In the external approach the break is closed by indenting the sclera with an externally located strip of silicone. This relieves the vitreous traction on the retinal hole and apposes the retinal pigment epithelium with the retina. It may first be necessary to drain an extensive accumulation of sub-retinal fluid by piercing the sclera and choroid with a needle (*sclerostomy*).

In the internal approach the vitreous is removed with a special microsurgical cutter introduced into the vitreous cavity through the pars plana, this relieves the vitreous traction on the break. Fluid can be drained

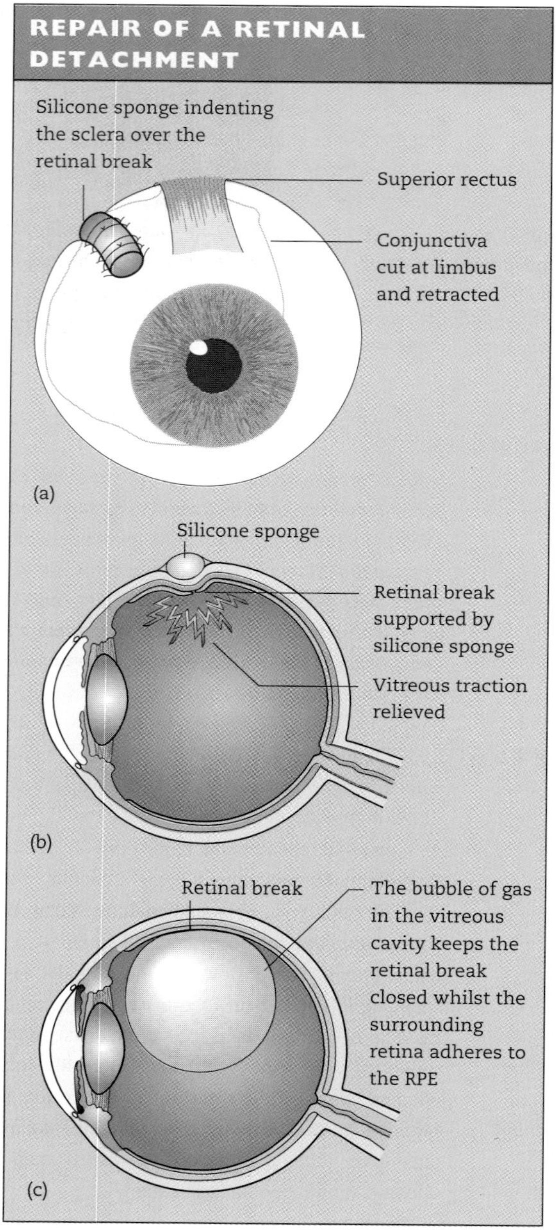

REPAIR OF A RETINAL DETACHMENT

Silicone sponge indenting the sclera over the retinal break

Superior rectus

Conjunctiva cut at limbus and retracted

(a)

Silicone sponge

Retinal break supported by silicone sponge

Vitreous traction relieved

(b)

Retinal break

The bubble of gas in the vitreous cavity keeps the retinal break closed whilst the surrounding retina adheres to the RPE

(c)

Fig. 11.10 The repair of a retinal detachment: (a) external approach, a silicone sponge has been sutured to the globe to indent the sclera over the retinal break following drainage of the sub-retinal fluid and application of cryotherapy; (b) sagittal section of the eye showing the indent formed by the silicone sponge, the retina is now reattached and traction on the retinal break by the vitreous is relieved; (c) internal approach, following removal of the vitreous gel and drainage of subretinal fluid an inert fluorocarbon gas has been injected into the vitreous cavity.

through the causative retinal break itself and laser or cryotherapy applied to the surrounding retina. A temporary internal tamponade is then obtained by injecting an inert fluorocarbon gas into the vitreous cavity. This has the effect of closing the hole from the inside and preventing further passage of fluid through the break. The patient has to maintain a particular head posture for a few days to ensure that the bubble continuously covers the retinal break.

Retinal tears may be found in undetached retina in fellow eyes of patients with retinal detachments. These are treated prophylactically with a laser or cryoprobe to induce inflammation and increase the adhesion between the surrounding retina and pigment epithelium.

PROGNOSIS

If the macula is attached and the surgery successfully reattaches the peripheral retina the outlook for vision is excellent. If the macula is detached for more than 24 hours prior to surgery the previous visual acuity will probably not be recovered. Nonetheless a substantial part of the vision may be restored over several months. If the retina is not successfully attached and the surgery is complicated, then fibrotic changes may occur in the vitreous (*proliferative vitreoretinopathy, PVR*). This may cause traction on the retina and further retinal detachment. A complex vitreoretinal procedure may permit vision to be retained but the outlook for vision is much poorer.

Traction retinal detachment

The retina is pulled away from the pigment epithelium by contracting fibrous tissue which has grown on the retinal surface. This may be seen in proliferative diabetic retinopathy or may occur as a result of proliferative vitreoretinopathy. Vitreoretinal surgery is required to repair these detachments.

INHERITED RETINAL DYSTROPHIES AND PHOTORECEPTOR DYSTROPHIES

Retinitis pigmentosa (Fig. 11.11)

Retinitis pigmentosa is an inherited disorder of the photoreceptors which has several genotypic and phenotypic varieties. It may occur in isolation or in association with a number of other systemic diseases.

PATHOGENESIS

The disease affects both types of photoreceptors but the rods are particularly affected. The inheritance may be:
- autosomal recessive (sporadic cases are often in this category);
- autosomal dominant;
- X-linked recessive.

Several forms of retinitis pigmentosa have been shown to be due to mutations in the gene for rhodopsin.

EPIDEMIOLOGY

The prevalence of this group of diseases is 1 in 4000.

SYMPTOMS

The age of onset, progression and prognosis is dependent on the mode of inheritance. In general the dominant form is of later onset and milder degree; recessive and X-linked recessive forms may present in infancy or childhood. Patients notice poor night vision, visual fields become increasingly constricted and central vision may ultimately be lost.

SIGNS

The three signs of typical retinitis pigmentosa are:

1 peripheral clumps of retinal pigmentation (termed 'bone-spicule' pigmentation);

2 attenuation of the retinal arterioles;

3 disc pallor.

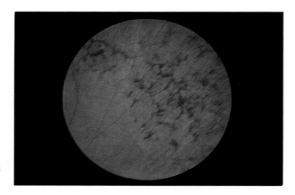

Fig. 11.11 The clinical appearance of the peripheral retina in retinitis pigmentosa.

Patients may also have cataracts at an early age and may develop macular oedema.

INVESTIGATION

A careful family history will help to determine the mode of inheritance. The diagnosis can usually be made clinically. Electrophysiologic tests are also useful in diagnosis, particularly in early disease where there may be few clinical signs.

Recent work on mapping the genetic loci for the condition has opened new avenues for genetic counselling and determining disease mechanism.

The possibility of associated syndromes should be borne in mind. Usher's syndrome, for example, is a recessive disorder characterised by deafness and retinitis pigmentosa. Retinitis pigmentosa also occurs in mitochondrial disease.

MANAGEMENT

Unfortunately nothing can be done to prevent the progression of the disease. Associated ocular problems can be treated. Cataracts can be removed and macular oedema may respond to treatment with acetazolamide. Low visual aids may be helpful for a period. The possibility of genetic counselling should be discussed with the patient.

PROGNOSIS

X-linked recessive and autosomal recessive disease produce the most severe visual symptoms. About 50% of all patients with retinitis pigmentosa will have an acuity of less than 6/60 by the time they reach 50.

Cone dystrophy

This is less common than retinitis pigmentosa. It is usually autosomal dominant but many cases are sporadic. Patients present in the first decade of life with poor vision. Examination reveals an abnormal, banded macular appearance which has been likened to a bull's-eye target. No treatment is possible but it is important to provide appropriate help not only to help maximize vision but also to help with educational problems. Genetic counselling should be offered.

JUVENILE MACULAR DYSTROPHIES

There are a variety of inherited conditions that affect both the retinal pigment epithelium and, secondarily, the photoreceptors. All are rare (e.g. the recessive disorder *Stargardt's dystrophy*) and the prognosis for vision is often poor. Once again the social and educational needs of the patient need to be assessed and genetic counselling offered.

ALBINISM

These patients have defective melanin synthesis. There are two types:

1 Ocular albinism where the lack of pigmentation is confined to the eye. There are X-linked and recessive forms.

2 Oculocutaneous albinism — a recessive disorder where the hair is white and the skin is pale; a few of these patients can manufacture some melanin.

Clinically the iris is blue and there is marked transillumination so that the red reflex is seen through the iris because of the lack of pigmentation, this also allows the lens edge to be viewed. The fundus appears abnormal, with lack of a normal foveal reflex, extreme pallor and prominent visibility of the choroidal vessels. Vision is poor from birth and the patients may have nystagmus. There is an abnormal projection of retinal axons to the lateral geniculate bodies.

Some patients will have associated systemic disease (e.g. the Hermansky–Pudlak syndrome where there is an associated haemorrhagic diathesis).

RETINAL TUMOURS

Retinoblastoma

This is the commonest malignant tumour of the eye in childhood with a frequency of 1 per 20 000 births. It may be inherited as an autosomal dominant condition but most cases are sporadic. These may be caused either by germinal mutations which can be passed on to the next generation or by somatic mutations (the majority, some 66% of cases) in a single retinal cell which cannot be genetically transmitted. The retinoblastoma gene has been located and the gene product is thought to control the differentiation of the retinal cell. The disease occurs when the individual has a homozygous defect in the retinoblastoma gene. In inherited retinoblastoma one gene error is inherited and the other occurs by spontaneous somatic mutation in the retina during development. The mutation rate for the gene is thought to be 1 : 10 000 000 and 100 000 000 divisions are needed to form the adult retina thus the chance of a somatic mutation occuring in a subject with only one functioning gene is very high. The homozygous state is thus achieved by a '*double hit*' event and the condition behaves as a *pseudodominant disorder*. Although it occurs frequently in affected families there may be some skip generations. Theoretically the disease should behave in a recessive fashion as only one functioning gene is required to control retinal cell differentiation.

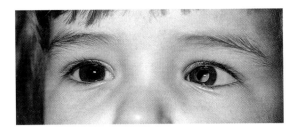

Fig. 11.12 Left leukocoria.

HISTORY AND SYMPTOMS

The child may present (at a mean age of 8 months if inherited and 25 months if sporadic) with:

- A white pupillary reflex (*leukocoria*) due to a pale elevated tumour at the posterior pole of the eye. Sometimes the tumour is bilateral on presentation (Fig. 11.12).
- A squint due to reduced vision.
- Occasionally, a painful red eye.

Most cases present by the age of two. Inherited retinoblastoma is often bilateral. When the condition is unilateral on presentation and there is no family history, inherited disease is less likely, but not excluded.

SIGNS

Dilated fundoscopy shows a whitish pink mass protruding from the retina into the vitreous cavity.

INVESTIGATIONS

The diagnosis is usually a clinical one. Cerebrospinal fluid and bone marrow must be examined to check for metastatic disease.

TREATMENT

Removal (enucleation) of the eye is performed in advanced cases. Radiotherapy can be used in less advanced disease as can cryotherapy and photocoagulation. Metastatic disease (either by direct spread through the optic nerve or by a haematogenous route) is treated with chemotherapy. Regular follow-up of an affected child is required and of subsequent offspring. Genetic counselling should be offered and children whose parents have had a retinoblastoma should be assessed from infancy.

PROGNOSIS

This depends on the extent of the disease at diagnosis. Overall the mortality of the condition is 15%. Unfortunately some 50% of children with the germinal mutation will develop a second primary tumour (e.g. an osteosarcoma of the femur) or a tumour related to treatment with radiotherapy.

Astrocytomas (Fig. 11.13)

These tumours of the retina and optic nerve are seen in patients with:
- tuberose sclerosis;
- neurofibromatosis (less commonly).

They appear as white berry-like lesions, are seldom symptomatic and require no treatment. However, their identification may assist in the diagnosis of important systemic disease.

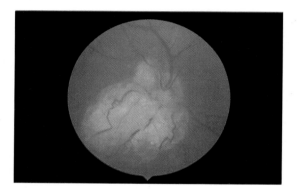

Fig. 11.13 The clinical appearance of a retinal astrocytoma.

CHOROIDAL TUMOURS

Melanoma (Fig. 11.14)

Pigmented fundus lesions include:
- retinal pigment hypertrophy;
- areas of old chorioretinitis;
- choroidal naevi;
- the rarest cause, a malignant melanoma.

Uveal melanomas have an incidence of 6 per 1 000 000 per year in white adults. It is seen very much more commonly in white than non-white races. It usually presents from middle-age onwards (40–70). Malignant melanoma may also be seen in the ciliary body and iris but by far the greatest number (80%) are found in the choroid.

SYMPTOMS

The presence of a melanoma may be detected as a coincidental finding during ocular examination. Advanced cases may present with a visual field defect or loss of acuity. If situated in the anterior part of the choroid the enlarging tumour may cause shallowing of the anterior chamber resulting in secondary angle closure glaucoma. In this country it is unusual for the tumour to be so advanced that it results in visible destruction of the eye.

SIGNS

A raised, usually pigmented, lesion is visible at the back of the eye, this may be associated with an area of retinal detachment. The optic nerve may be involved.

INVESTIGATIONS

The patient is investigated for systemic spread although this is less usual than in malignant melanoma of the skin. An ultrasound of the eye is useful in determining the size of the tumour and can be used both for quantative assessment and in detecting the growth of tumours over time.

TREATMENT

A number of therapies are available. The treatment used depends on the size and location of the tumour. Large tumours that have reduced vision, or are close to the optic nerve, usually require removal of the eye (enucleation). Smaller tumours can be treated by:

• local excision;
• local radiation applied to the lesion by an overlying radioactive plaque;
• proton beam irradiation.

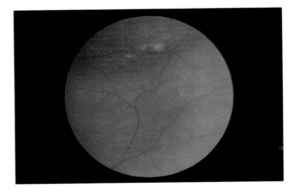

Fig. 11.14 The clinical appearance of a choroidal melanoma.

PROGNOSIS

This depends very much on the type of tumour (some are more rapidly growing than others) and its location (tumours involving the sclera and optic nerve carry a poorer prognosis). The existence of metastatic lesions at the time of diagnosis carries a poor prognosis. Some tumours are very slow growing and have an excellent prognosis. Others, which extend into the optic nerve or through the sclera, are more malignant and result in secondary spread.

Metastatic tumours

These account for the greater part of ocular malignant disease. In women the commonest site of spread is from the breast, in men the commonest source is the bronchus. Symptoms and signs depend on their location in the eye. They appear as a whitish lesion with little elevation, and may be multiple. Treatment is usually by external beam radiotherapy.

KEY POINTS

- A curtain like partial loss of vision suggests a retinal detachment and requires urgent ophthalmic assessment.
- Distortion of vision is a sign of macular disease.
- Age-related macular degeneration results in loss of acuity but never total loss of vision.
- Children with a white pupil require urgent ophthalmic investigation.

Box 11.1 Key points in retinal disease.

CHAPTER 12

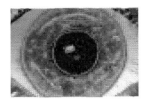

Retinal vascular disease

INTRODUCTION

The eye is an organ in which much of the microcirculation is readily visualized. Vascular disease affecting the eye can thus be seen directly. Furthermore the eye provides important clues about pathological vascular changes in the rest of the body.

SIGNS OF RETINAL VASCULAR DISEASE
(Figs. 12.1 & 12.2)

The signs of retinal vascular disease result from two changes to the retinal capillary circulation:
- leakage from the microcirculation;
- occlusion of the microcirculation.

Leakage from the microcirculation

This results in:
- *haemorrhages* caused by leakage of blood from damaged vessels;
- *oedema* of the retina, the result of fluid leakage from damaged vessels;
- *exudates* formed by lipids, lipoprotein and lipid containing macrophages. These are yellow in colour, with well-defined margins.

Occlusion of the microcirculation

This results in:

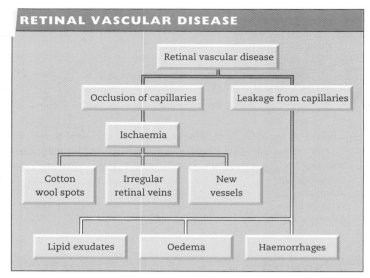

Fig. 12.1 Diagram showing the building blocks of retinal vascular disease.

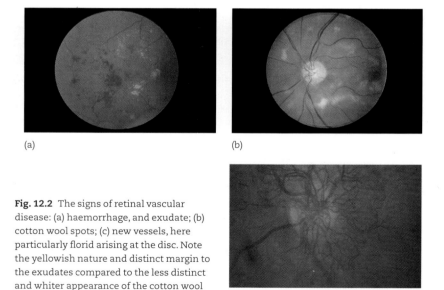

(a)

(b)

Fig. 12.2 The signs of retinal vascular disease: (a) haemorrhage, and exudate; (b) cotton wool spots; (c) new vessels, here particularly florid arising at the disc. Note the yellowish nature and distinct margin to the exudates compared to the less distinct and whiter appearance of the cotton wool spot.

(c)

- *Cotton wool spots* (previously termed *soft exudates*). These are caused by a build-up of axonal debris in the nerve fibre layer of the retina. This results from a hold-up in axoplasmic transport due to ischaemia. Cotton wool spots are found at the margins of ischaemic infarcts. Their visibility depends on nerve fibre layer thickness so that they are seen close to the optic disc, where the nerve fibre layer is thick, and not in the periphery where the nerve fibre layer is thin. They are white in colour with indistinct borders.
- *New vessels.* Ischaemic retina release vasogenic factors which result in the growth of abnormal blood vessels and fibrous tissue onto the retinal surface and forward into the vitreous. These intravitreal vessels are much more permeable than normal retinal vessels, and their abnormal position predisposes them to break and bleed.

The diseases affecting the vasculature of the eye may be classified as shown in Box 12.1.

OCULAR CIRCULATION

Diabetic retinopathy
Central retinal artery occlusion
Branch retinal artery occlusion
Central retinal vein occlusion
Branch retinal vein occlusion
Ischaemic optic neuropathy
Hypertensive retinopathy
Retinopathy of prematurity
Sickle cell retinopathy
Abnormal retinal blood vessels

Box 12.1 Classification of disease affecting the ocular circulation.

DIABETIC RETINOPATHY (Fig. 12.3)

Diabetes results from a defect in both insulin secretion and action leading to hyperglycaemia.

EPIDEMIOLOGY

In the UK diabetic eye disease is the commonest reason for blind registration in the 30–65 age group.

Type 1 diabetes (eventual loss of insulin secretion, mostly in young people with associated HLA types) has a prevalence in the UK of 2 per 1000 under the age of 20.

Type II diabetes (a heterogeneous group of patients with familial aggregation, usually with some insulin secretion remaining but with the development of resistance to insulin, occurring in an older age group) has a prevalence of 5–20 per 1000.

Diabetes is associated with the following ocular events:
- retinopathy;
- specific cataract types and the earlier onset of age related cataract;
- glaucoma (but the association with chronic open angle glaucoma is disputed);
- extraocular muscle palsy due to microvascular disease of the third, fourth, or sixth cranial nerves.

PATHOLOGY

Factors thought to be important in the development of diabetic retinopathy include:
- The length of time that the patient has had diabetes (patients who have had the disease for 20 years have an 80% chance of having retinopathy).
- Diabetic control.
- Coexisting diseases particularly hypertension.
- Smoking (possibly).

The development of retinopathy may also be accelerated by pregnancy and patients require careful screening.

Retinal damage results from damage to the circulation. Pathological studies show that there is a:
- decrease in the number of pericytes surrounding the capillary endothelium;
- development of microaneurysms on the capillary network which allow plasma to leak out into the retina;
- development of arterio-venous shunts with closure of the capillary net resulting in areas of ischaemic retina.

HISTORY

Diabetic retinopathy should ideally be diagnosed before it is symptomatic. All diabetics should have fundoscopy performed at least yearly. Visual acuity may be reduced gradually by a maculopathy and suddenly from a vitreous haemorrhage.

EXAMINATION

The building blocks of the disease are those of leakage and microvascular occlusion discussed earlier. The classification of retinopathy is shown in Table 12.1.

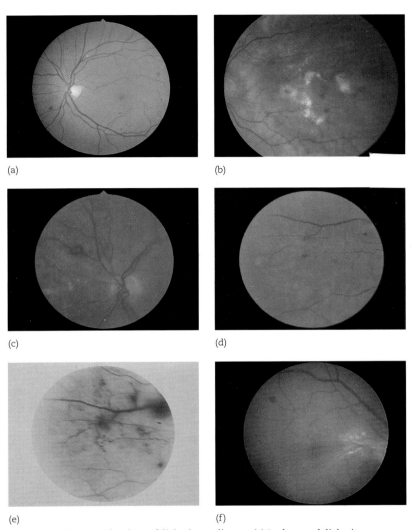

(a)

(b)

(c)

(d)

(e)

(f)

Fig. 12.3 The signs of diabetic eye disease. (a) Background diabetic retinopathy. (b) Diabetic maculopathy, note the circinate exudate temporal to the macula. (c) Preproliferative retinopathy with a venous loop. (d, e) Proliferative retinopathy. New vessels have formed on the retina, their presence is demonstrated by leakage of fluorescein (hyperfluorescence) on the fluorescein angiogram. Closure of some of the retinal capillary network is demonstrated by its failure to fill with fluorescein. (f) Advanced diabetic retinopathy, the neovascularisation has caused a traction retinal detachment.

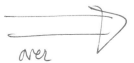

DIABETIC RETINOPATHY

Stage	Description
No retinopathy	There are no abnormal signs present on the retina. *Vision normal*
Background	Signs of microvascular leakage (haemorrhage and exudates) away from the macula. *Vision normal*
Maculopathy	Exudates and haemorrhages within the macula region, and/or evidence of retinal oedema, and/or evidence of retinal ischaemia. *Vision may be reduced, sight threatening*
Preproliferative	Evidence of occlusion (cotton wool spots). The veins become irregular and may show loops. *Vision normal*
Proliferative	The occlusive changes have led to the release of a vasoproliferative substance from the retina resulting in the growth of new vessels either on the disc (NVD) or elsewhere on the retina (NVE). *Vision normal, sight threatening*
Advanced	The proliferative changes may result in bleeding into the vitreous or between the vitreous and the retina. The retina may also be pulled from its underlying pigment epithelium by a fibrous proliferation associated with the growth of the new vessels. *Vision reduced, often acutely with vitreous haemorrhage, sight threatening*

Table 12.1 The classification of diabetic retinopathy (note that diabetic maculopathy may coexist with other stages in the classification).

CLINICAL OBSERVATIONS

- Younger patients are more likely to develop proliferative disease.
- Older patients more commonly develop a maculopathy but because type II disease is more common, it is also an important cause of proliferative disease.

Box 12.2 Clinical observations.

TREATMENT

Patients with a maculopathy, preproliferative or proliferative retinopathy or worse require referral to an ophthalmologist. Any patient with unexplained visual loss should also be referred. The mainstay of treatment for sight threatening diabetic retinopathy is the laser. A fluorescein angiogram may be performed in some patients to assess the degree of retinal ischaemia and to pinpoint areas of leakage both from microaneurysms and new vessels.

Laser treatment of both the maculopathy and new vessels can be performed on an outpatient basis.

• Diabetic maculopathy is treated by aiming the laser at the points of leakage. The exudate is often seen to be in a circinate pattern with the focus of leakage or microaneurysm in the middle. If effective the retinal oedema and exudate will resorb although this may take some months.

• Optic disc and retinal new vessels are treated with scattered laser burns to the entire retina leaving an untreated area around the macula and optic disc (Fig. 12.4). The laser treatment eliminates ischaemic retina thus preventing the release of vasoproliferative factors. This results in the regression of the new vessels thus preventing the development of advanced retinopathy.

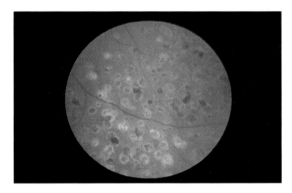

Fig. 12.4 Typical appearance of retinal laser burns.

The development of vitreous haemorrhage which does not clear after a few months or fibrous traction on the retina causing detachment from the underlying pigment epithelium (tractional retinal detachment) may require surgical treatment. A vitrectomy is performed to remove the vitreous gel and blood and repair any of the detached retina.

PROGNOSIS

Although laser and surgical treatments have greatly improved the prognosis of patients with diabetic retinopathy the disease may still cause severe visual loss in some patients.

ARTERIAL OCCLUSION

PATHOGENESIS

Central and branch retinal artery occlusions are usually embolic in origin. Three types of emboli are recognized:

1 *fibrin-platelet* emboli commonly from diseased carotid arteries;

2 *cholesterol* emboli commonly from diseased carotid arteries (Fig. 12.5);

3 *calcific* emboli from diseased heart valves.

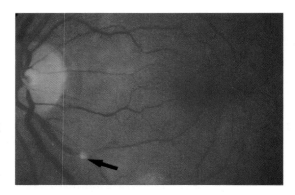

Fig. 12.5 The clinical appearance of a cholesterol embolus (arrow). They appear to sparkle when viewed with a direct ophthalmoscope.

HISTORY

The patient complains of a sudden painless loss of all or part of the vision. Fibrin platelet emboli typically cause a fleeting loss of vision as the emboli passes through the retinal circulation (*amaurosis fugax*). This may last for some minutes and then clears. Cholesterol and calcific emboli may result in permanent obstruction with no recovery in vision (they may also be seen in the retinal vessels of asymptomatic individuals). A central retinal artery obstruction is frequently caused by an embolus, although as it lodges further back in the arterial tree behind the optic nerve head, it cannot be seen.

In young patients episodes of amaurosis fugax may be caused by migraine.

SIGNS

Occasionally, a series of white platelet emboli can be seen passing rapidly through a vessel; more often a bright yellow, reflective cholesterol embolus is noted occluding an arterial branch point. The acutely affected retina is swollen and white (*oedematous*), while the fovea is red (*cherry red spot*) as it has no supply from the retinal circulation, is not swollen, and the normal choroid can be seen through it. After several weeks the disc becomes pale (*atrophic*) and the arterioles attenuated. The condition may also occasionally be caused by vasculitis, such as giant cell arteritis (see p. 155).

INVESTIGATION

Patients require a careful vascular work-up since disease in the eye may reflect systemic vascular disease. A search for carotid artery disease should be made by assessing the strength of carotid pulsation and listening for bruits. Ischaemic heart disease, peripheral claudication and hypertension may also be present.

A carotid endarterectomy may be indicated to prevent the possibility of a cerebral embolus if a stenosis of the carotid artery greater than 75% is present. Doppler ultrasound allows non-invasive imaging of both the carotid and vertebral arteries to detect such a stenosis.

TREATMENT

Acute treatment of central and branch artery occlusions is aimed at dilating the arteriole to permit the embolus to pass more distally. Results are usually disappointing although a trial is worthwhile if the patient is seen within 24 hours of onset of the obstruction. The patient is referred to an eye unit where the following measures may be tried:

*   lowering the intraocular pressure with intravenous acetazolamide;
*   ocular massage;
*   paracentesis (a needle is inserted into the anterior chamber to allow aqueous to pass out of the eye rapidly lowering the intraocular pressure);
*   getting the patient to rebreath into a paper bag firmly applied around the mouth and nose to use the vasodilatatory effect of raised carbon dioxide levels.

PROGNOSIS

Full visual recovery occurs with amaurosis fugax but more prolonged arterial occlusion results in severe unrecoverable visual loss.

VENOUS OCCLUSION (Fig. 12.6)

PATHOGENESIS

Central retinal vein occlusion (CRVO) may result from:

*   abnormality of the blood itself (the hyperviscosity syndromes and abnormalities in coagulation);
*   an abnormality of the venous wall (inflammation);
*   an increased ocular pressure.

HISTORY

The patient complains of a sudden partial or complete loss of vision.

SIGNS

These contrast markedly with those of arterial occlusion. There is marked haemorrhage and great tortuosity and swelling of the veins. The optic disc appears swollen. Branch retinal vein occlusion may originate at the crossing point of an arteriole and a vein where the arteriole has been affected by arteriosclerosis associated with hypertension.

Subsequently:

• Abnormal new vessels may grow on the retina and optic disc causing vitreous haemorrhage. This happens if the retina has become ischaemic as a result of the vein occlusion (an ischaemic retinal vein occlusion).

• In ischaemic retinal vein occlusion abnormal new vessels may grow on the iris causing rubeotic glaucoma.

INVESTIGATION

Investigation of a CRVO includes vascular and haematological work up to exclude increased blood viscosity. Central retinal vein occlusion is also associated with raised ocular pressure, diabetes and hypertension.

TREATMENT

Retinal laser treatment is given if the retina is ischaemic to prevent the development of retinal and iris new vessels (see glaucoma). Laser treatment may improve vision in some patients with a branch retinal vein occlusion by reducing retinal oedema.

PROGNOSIS

The vision is usually severely affected in central, and often in branch, vein occlusion and usually does not improve. Younger patients may fare better, and there may well be some visual improvement.

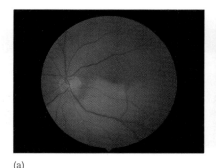
(a)

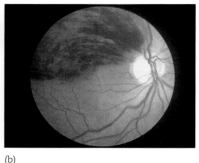
(b)

Fig. 12.6 The contrast between: (a) an inferior branch retinal artery occlusion (note the white appearance of the affected retina) and; (b) a superior branch vein occlusion.

ARTERIOSCLEROSIS AND HYPERTENSION

Arteriosclerosis can be visualized in the eye as an attenuation of the retinal arterial vessels (sometimes referred to as *copper* and *silver wiring*) and by the presence of nipping of the retinal vein where it is crossed by an arteriole. Hypertension may cause a breakdown in the blood retinal barrier resulting in the signs of vascular leakage (haemorrhage and exudate). These are particularly prominent if the hypertension is of renal origin. If severe the retina may also demonstrate signs of capillary occlusion (cotton wool spots). Very high blood pressure may cause swelling of the optic disc as well as these other signs (*malignant hypertension*; Fig. 12.7). The patient may complain of blurring of vision and episodes of temporary visual loss, though severe retinopathy may also be asymptomatic.

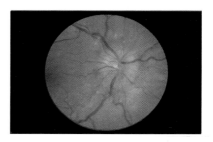

Fig. 12.7 The fundus in malignant hypertension. The disc is swollen, there are retinal haemorrhages and exudates.

Treatment of the hypertension, avoiding a rapid reduction which may precipitate vascular occlusion, results in the resolution of the retinal signs. This may take some months.

RETINOPATHY OF PREMATURITY

PATHOGENESIS

There is an initial failure of normal retinal vascularization followed by a phase of aggressive new vessel formation extending forward into the vitreous and causing traction detachment.

Risk factors associated with retinopathy of prematurity include:
- gestation less than 32 weeks;
- birth weight below 1500 g;
- exposure to supplemental oxygen;
- apnoea;
- sepsis;
- duration of ventilation;
- blood transfusion;
- the presence of intraventricular haemorrhage;

- retinal light exposure.

The incidence of the condition in infants weighing less than 1500 g is between 34–60%.

SIGNS

The retinal appearance depends on the severity of the condition but includes:

- new vessels;
- the development of retinal haemorrhage;
- increased tortuosity and dilation of the retinal vessels.

In severe disease:

- bleeding into the vitreous;
- retinal detachment;
- blindness.

TREATMENT

At-risk infants are screened on a regular basis. The severe complications of the condition can be reduced by applying cryotherapy or argon laser to the avascular retina.

HT   LE CELL RETINOPATHY

Patients with sickle cell haemoglobin C disease (SC disease) and sickle cell haemoglobin with thalassaemia (SThal) develop a severe form of retinopathy. This is unusual in homozygous sickle cell disease (SS) where the retinopathy is more confined. Signs include:

- tortuous veins;
- peripheral haemorrhages;
- capillary non-perfusion;
- pigmented spots on the retina;
- new vessel formation, classically in a 'sea-fan' pattern, which may occur as a result of peripheral retinal artery occlusion.

New vessels may cause vitreous haemorrhage and traction retinal detachment. As with diabetes this may require treatment with laser photocoagulation and vitrectomy.

ABNORMAL RETINAL BLOOD VESSELS

Abnormality of the retinal blood vessels may be seen in rare ocular diseases where they are associated with the development of massive exudate. They may also be an indication of systemic disorders as in the retinal and optic disc angioma associated with the familial von Hippel-

Lindau syndrome. Here the ocular condition may be associated with angioma in the brain and spinal cord. Patients and their relatives require repeated MRI screening.

ABNORMALITIES OF THE BLOOD

Clotting abnormalities may be responsible for occlusion of any blood vessel in the eye (e.g. a central retinal vein occlusion). Similarly increased viscosity may also cause vessel occlusion. Leukaemia with a greatly raised white cell count may lead to the development of a haemorrhagic retinopathy in which the haemorrhages have white centres (*Roth spots*) (Fig. 12.8). These may also be a feature of bacterial endocarditis and autoimmune diseases associated with vasculitis.

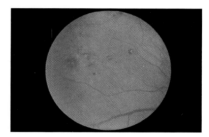

Fig. 12.8 White centred haemorrhages.

KEY POINTS

- Premature infants require screening for retinopathy of prematurity.
- Diabetics require regular screening for sight-threatening retinopathy.

Box 12.3 Key points in retinal vascular disease.

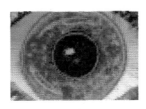

The pupil

INTRODUCTION

Movements of the pupil are controlled by the parasympathetic and sympathetic nervous systems. The pupils constrict (*miosis*) when the eye is illuminated (parasympathetic activation, sympathetic relaxation) and dilate (*mydriasis*) in the dark (sympathetic activation, parasympathetic relaxation). When the eyes accommodate the eyes converge and the pupils constrict. The pupils are normally equal in size but some 20% of people may have noticeably unequal pupils (*anisocoria*) with no associated disease. The key to diagnosis of pupillary disorders is to:
- determine which pupil is abnormal;
- search for associated signs.

   Disorders of the pupil may result from:
- ocular disease;
- disorders of the controlling neurological pathway;
- pharmacological action.

   The parasympathetic fibres reach the eye through the third cranial nerve. The sympathetic pathway is shown in Fig. 13.1.

OCULAR CAUSES OF PUPILLARY ABNORMALITY

Diseases of the eye which cause irregularity of the pupil and alter its reaction, include:
- ocular inflammation where posterior synechiae give the pupil an irregular appearance (see p. 90);
- the sequelae of intraocular surgery;

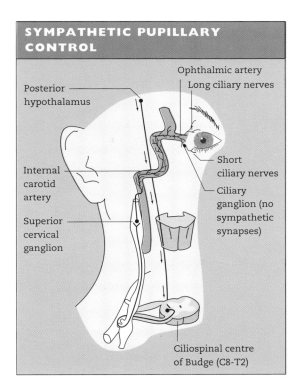

SYMPATHETIC PUPILLARY CONTROL

Posterior hypothalamus

Ophthalmic artery

Long ciliary nerves

Internal carotid artery

Superior cervical ganglion

Short ciliary nerves

Ciliary ganglion (no sympathetic synapses)

Ciliospinal centre of Budge (C8-T2)

Fig. 13.1 The pathway of sympathetic pupillary control. (With permission from Kanski JJ (1994) *Clinical Ophthalmology.* Butterworth-Heinemann, Oxford).

- blunt trauma to the eye which may rupture the sphincter muscle causing irregularity, or fixed dilation (*traumatic mydriasis*).

NEUROLOGICAL CAUSES OF AN ABNORMAL PUPIL

Horner's syndrome (Fig. 13.2)

Interruption of the sympathetic pathway causes:
- A small pupil on the affected side. This is more noticeable in the dark when the fellow, normal pupil, dilates more than the affected pupil.
- A slight ptosis on the affected side.
- Lack of sweating on the affected side if the sympathetic pathway is affected proximal to the base of the skull.
- An apparent recession of the globe into the orbit.

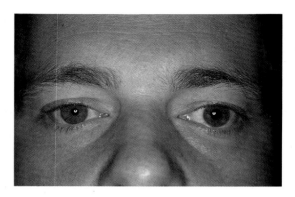

Fig. 13.2 A right ptosis and miosis in Horner's syndrome.

Because of its extended course the sympathetic pathway may be affected by a multitude of pathologies. Examples include:
- Syringomyelia, a cavity within the spinal cord sometimes extending into the medulla (syringobulbia). Typically it also causes wasting of the hand muscles and loss of sensation.
- Disease of the lung apex (e.g. neoplasia). Involvement of the brachial plexus gives rise to pain and to T1-wasting of the small muscles of the hand, in Pancoast's syndrome.
- Neck injury, disease or surgery.
- Cavernous sinus disease.

Horner's syndrome may also be congenital. Here the iris colour may be altered when compared to the fellow eye (*heterochromia*).

LIGHT-NEAR DISSOCIATION

In these pupillary abnormalities the reaction of the pupils to light is much less than to the near (accommodative) response. There is no condition in which the light reflex is intact but the near reflex is defective. A light-near dissociation is seen in diabetes and multiple sclerosis or may be caused by periaqueductal brainstem lesions (see below).

Relative afferent pupillary defect

A lesion of the optic nerve on one side blocks the afferent limb of the pupillary light reflex (see p. 25). The pupils are equal and of normal size, but the pupillary response to light on the affected side is reduced, while the near reflex is intact. This is an important test to perform in a patient suspected of having an optic nerve lesion, such as optic neuritis. It may also, however, be seen in severe disease of the retina. It will not be seen in opacities of the cornea or lens.

Adie's pupil

This is not an unusual cause of unequal pupil size (*anisocoria*). It affects young adults and is seen more commonly in females than males (2 : 1). It is due to a ciliary ganglionitis which denervates the iris and ciliary body. Parasympathetic fibres which reinnervate the iris sphincter are those which were previously involved in accommodation. The affected pupil:

- Is enlarged.
- Is poorly reactive to light. On the slit lamp the pupil movement in response to light is seen as a worm-like (*vermiform*) contraction.
- Shows slow miosis on accommodation.
- Is supersensitive to dilute pilocarpine (0.1%).

The ability to accommodate is also impaired, the patient may complain of blurred vision when looking from a distant object to a near one and vice versa. Systemically the disorder is associated with loss of tendon reflexes; there are no other neurological signs.

Argyll Robertson pupil

Classically seen in neurosyphilis the pupils are bilaterally small and irregular. They do not react to light but do to accommodation. The iris stroma has a typical feathery appearance and loses its architectural detail.

Midbrain pupil

A lesion in the region of the pretectal nuclear complex disrupts retinotectal fibres but preserves the supranuclear accommodative pathway, causing mydriasis and light-near dissociation. These are usually seen as part of the *periaqueductal* (*Parinaud's*) syndrome (see p. 178).

Other causes of pupillary abnormality

In coma, both pupils may become miosed but remember that patients taking pilocarpine for glaucoma or receiving morphine also show bilateral miosis. Coma associated with a unilateral expanding supratentorial mass, e.g. a haematoma, results in pressure on the third nerve and dilation of the pupil. Intrinsic third nerve lesions also cause a dilated pupil (see p. 170). The pupil may also be affected by drugs, both topical and systemic (Table 13.1).

DRUGS AFFECTING THE PUPIL		
Action	**Mechanism**	**Agent**
Topical Agents		
Dilates	Muscarinic blockade	Cyclopentolate Tropicamide Atropine (long acting)
	Alpha-adrenergic Agonists	Phenylephrine Adrenaline Dipivefrin
Constricts	Muscarinic agonist	Pilocarpine
Systemic		
Dilates	Muscarinic blockade Alpha-adrenergic agonist	Atropine Adrenaline
Constricts	Local action and action on central nervous system	Morphine

Table 13.1 Drugs having a pharmacological effect on the pupil.

KEY POINTS
• Take a good history to help exclude an ocular cause for the pupillary changes and to see if a medical condition exists which may contribute to the pupillary problem. • Determine whether it is the small or the large pupil that is abnormal. • Search for associated signs that may help make a diagnosis.

Box 13.1 Key points in the assessment of abnormal pupils.

CHAPTER 14

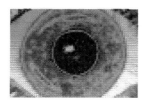

The visual pathway

INTRODUCTION

The innermost layer of the retina consists of the nerve fibres originating from its ganglion cells. These fibres collect together at the optic nerve head, and form the optic nerve (see p. 13). The subsequent course of the visual pathway is shown in the diagram. Diagnosis and location of disease of the optic pathways is greatly aided by the differing field defects produced, as Fig. 14.1 shows.

THE OPTIC NERVE

The normal optic nerve head has distinct margins, a pinkish rim and usually a white central cup. The central retinal artery and vein enter the globe slightly nasally in the optic nerve head. The optic disc may be involved in many disorders but has a limited repertoire of responses. Ophthalmoscopically it may become swollen, or it may become pale.

The swollen optic disc (Fig. 14.2)

The swollen disc is an important and often worrying sign. *Papilloedema* is the term given to disc swelling associated with raised intracranial pressure, accelerated hypertension and optic disc ischaemia. Optic neuritis affecting the nerve head (*papillitis*) has a similar appearance. The differential diagnosis of disc swelling is shown in Table 14.1.

Note also that *myelinated nerve fibres* (a normal variant where the normally unmyelinated retinal nerve fibre layer is partly myelinated giving it a white appearance) may be mistaken for optic disc swelling. A high myope

VISUAL PATHWAY

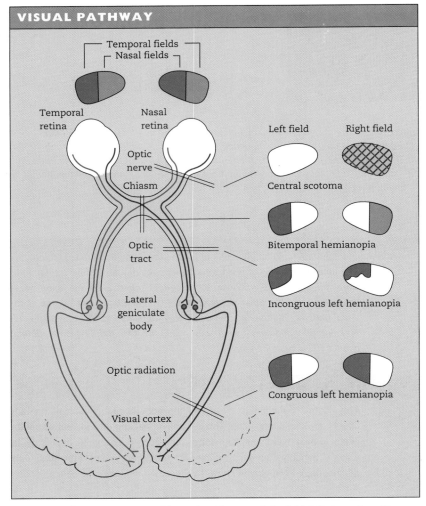

Fig. 14.1 Anatomy of the optic pathway and the field defects produced by lesions at different sites.

CAUSES OF A SWOLLEN OPTIC DISC

Condition	Distinguishing Features
Raised Intracranial Pressure	Vision and field usually normal save for large blind spot. *Obscurations* (short episodes of visual loss usually on changing posture). Field may be contracted in chronic disease. Colour vision normal. No RAPD. No spontaneous venous pulsation of the vein at the disc. (but some people with normal intracranial pressure do not have this). Dilated capillaries and haemorrhages on disc. Other symptoms and signs of raised intracranial pressure.
Space occupying lesions of the optic nerve head	Various solid, or infiltrative lesions at the nerve head, e.g. optic disc drusen (calcified axonal material), gliomas, sarcoidosis and leukaemia, may produce disc swelling. These may be associated with reduced and field defects.
Papillitis (Optic neuritis affecting the optic nerve head)	A swollen optic disc. Exudates around the macula may occasionally be seen. Vision is profoundly reduced. Colour vision is abnormal. RAPD present. A central field defect is present.
Accelerated (malignant) hypertension (see vascular eye disease)	Reduced vision, haemorrhagic disc swelling. Retinal haemorrhages, exudates and cotton wool spots away from the nerve head. Check blood pressure!
Ischaemic optic neuropathy —*may be. non arteritic*	Sudden visual loss, field defect. Colour vision may be normal. RAPD may be present. Spontaneous venous pulsation at the optic disc may be present. May be sectorial swelling only. Haemorrhages on disc and disc margin. Cotton wool spots may be seen around disc particularly if caused by giant cell arteritis.
Central retinal vein occlusion (see vascular eye disease)	Sudden marked visual loss, tortuous veins, gross retinal haemorrhage.

Table 14.1 Causes of a swollen optic disc (RAPD, relative afferent pupillary defect see p. 26).

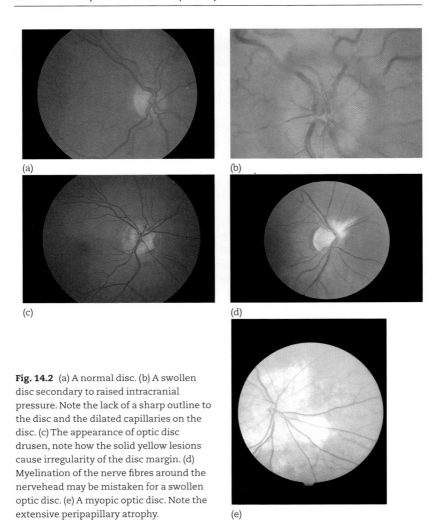

(a)

(b)

(c)

(d)

Fig. 14.2 (a) A normal disc. (b) A swollen disc secondary to raised intracranial pressure. Note the lack of a sharp outline to the disc and the dilated capillaries on the disc. (c) The appearance of optic disc drusen, note how the solid yellow lesions cause irregularity of the disc margin. (d) Myelination of the nerve fibres around the nervehead may be mistaken for a swollen optic disc. (e) A myopic optic disc. Note the extensive peripapillary atrophy.

(e)

may also have an optic disc surrounded by an atrophic area (*peripapillary atrophy*) that may be confused with disc swelling.

Papilloedema due to raised intracranial pressure

HISTORY

The crucial feature of disc swelling due to raised intracranial pressure is that there is no acute prolonged visual loss. Some patients may develop fleeting visual loss lasting seconds when they alter posture (*obscurations* of vision). Other features of raised intracranial pressure may be present including:

- headache, worse on waking and made worse by coughing;
- nausea, retching;
- diplopia (double vision) usually due to a sixth nerve palsy;
- neurological symptoms, if the raised pressure is due to a cranial space occupying lesion;
- a history of head trauma suggesting a subdural haemorrhage.

SIGNS

- The optic disc is swollen, the edges blurred and the superficial capillaries are dilated and thus abnormally prominent. There is no spontaneous venous pulsation of the central retinal vein (5–20% of those with normal nerve heads have no spontaneous pulsation, however).
- A large blind spot will be found on visual field testing corresponding to the increased size of the optic nerve head due to swelling. In chronic papilloedema the field may become constricted. A field defect may, however, be caused by the space-occupying lesion causing the papilloedema.
- Abnormal neurological signs may indicate the site of a space-occupying lesion.

INVESTIGATION

CT and MRI scanning will identify any space occupying lesion or enlargement of the ventricles. Following neurological consultation (and normally after a scan) a lumbar puncture will enable intracranial pressure to be measured.

TREATMENT

Intracranial pressure may be elevated and disc swelling present with no evidence of intracranial abnormality and no dilation of the ventricles on the scan. This is termed *benign intracranial hypertension* and usually presents in overweight women in the second and third decade. Patients complain of headache and may have obscurations of vision and sixth nerve palsies. No other neurological problems are present. Although acute permanent visual loss is not a feature of papilloedema, if the nerve remains swollen for several weeks there will be a progressive contraction of the visual field. It is thus important to reduce intracranial pressure. This may be achieved:

- with medications such as oral acetazolamide;
- through ventriculoperitoneal shunting;
- through optic nerve decompression where a small hole is made in the

sheath surrounding the optic nerve to allow the drainage of CSF and reduce the pressure of CSF around the anterior optic nerve.

Space-occupying lesions (i.e. tumours and haemorrhage) and hydro-cephalus require neurosurgical management.

Optic neuritis

Inflammation or demyelination of the optic nerve results in optic neuritis (termed *papillitis* if the optic nerve head is affected and *retrobulbar neuritis* if the optic nerve is affected more posteriorly).

HISTORY

There is:
- An acute loss of vision that may progress over a few days and then slowly improve.
- Pain on eye movement in retrobulbar neuritis because rectus contraction pulls on the optic nerve sheaf.
- A preceding history of viral illness in some cases. Between 40 and 70% of patients with optic neuritis will have or develop other neurological symptoms to suggest a diagnosis of demyelination (multiple sclerosis).

EXAMINATION

This reveals:
- reduced visual acuity;
- reduced colour vision;
- relative afferent pupillary defect (RAPD) (see p. 26);
- central scotoma on field testing;
- a normal disc in retrobulbar neuritis. A swollen disc in papillitis.

TREATMENT

There is usually no indication for any medical intervention except to diagnose a possible cause for the neuritis. An MRI scan will help to identify additional 'silent' plaques of demyelination but the patient must be suitably counselled before a scan is performed. In bilateral cases there may be a role for intravenous steroid treatment to speed up visual recovery (oral treatment has been shown to *increase* the number of episodes of optic neuritis).

PROGNOSIS

Vision slowly recovers over several weeks although often it is not quite as good as before the attack. Repeated episodes may lead to a decline in vision and optic atrophy.

Ischaemic optic neuropathy (Fig. 14.3)

PATHOGENESIS

The anterior optic nerve may become ischaemic if the posterior ciliary vessels are compromized as a result of degenerative or vasculitic disease of the arterioles (see p. 14). This results in an *anterior ischaemic optic neuropathy*.

SYMPTOMS

The patient complains of a sudden loss of vision or visual field, often on waking since vascular perfusion to the eye is decreased during sleep. If accompanied by pain or scalp tenderness the diagnosis of *giant cell arteritis* must never be forgotten. Ischaemic optic neuropathy is the usual cause of blindness in the disease.

Giant cell arteritis

This is an auto-immune disease occuring in patients generally over the age of 60. It affects arteries with an internal elastic lamina. It may present with any combination of:
- sudden loss of vision;
- scalp tenderness;
- pain on chewing (*jaw claudication*);
- shoulder pain;
- malaise.

SIGNS

There is usually:
- A reduction in visual acuity.
- A field defect, typically an absence of the lower half of the visual field.
- A swollen and haemorrhagic disc with normal retina and retinal vessels (remember the blood supply to the anterior optic nerve and retina are different). In arteritic ischaemic optic neuropathy the disc may be pale.
- A small fellow disc with a small cup in non-arteritic disease.
- A tender temporal artery, a sign suggestive of giant cell arteritis.

INVESTIGATIONS

If giant cell arteritis is present the ESR and C-reactive protein are usually grossly elevated (although 1 in 10 patients with giant cell arteritis have a normal ESR). Temporal artery biopsy is often helpful but again may not lead to a diagnosis, particularly if only a small specimen is examined, because the disease may skip a length of the artery. Giant cell arteritis can also present as a central retinal artery occlusion when the vessel is affected secondary to arteritis of the ophthalmic artery.

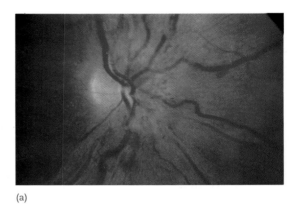

(a)

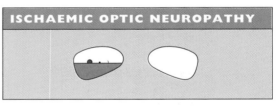

(b)

Fig. 14.3 The clinical appearance of the optic disc and one form of field defect (attitudinal) seen in ischaemic optic neuropathy.

Investigation of the patient with non-arteritic ischaemic optic neuropathy includes:
- a full blood count to exclude anaemia;
- blood pressure check;
- blood sugar check;
- ESR and C-reactive protein to check for giant cell arteritis.

Both hypertension and diabetes may be associated with the condition. It may also be seen in patients suffering acute blood loss, e.g. haematemesis, where it may occur some days after the acute bleed. Hypotensive episodes may also give rise to ischaemic optic neuropathy. Occasionally clotting disorders or autoimmune disease may cause the condition.

TREATMENT

If giant cell arteritis is suspected treatment must not be delayed while the diagnosis is confirmed. High-dose steroids must be given, intravenously and orally, and the dose tapered over the ensuing weeks according to both symptoms and the response of the ESR or C-reactive protein. The usual precautions must be taken, as with any patient on steroids, to exclude other medical conditions that might be unmasked or made worse by the steroids (e.g. tuberculosis, diabetes, hypertension and an increased susceptiblity to infection). Steroids will not reverse the visual loss but should help prevent the fellow eye being affected.

There is unfortunately no treatment for non-arteritic ischaemic optic neuropathy other than the diagnosis of underlying conditions.

PROGNOSIS

It is unusual for the vision to get progressively worse and the visual outcome both in terms of visual field and acuity is very variable. Vision is not recovered once it has been lost. The second eye may rapidly become involved in patients with untreated giant cell arteritis. There is also a significant rate of involvement of the second eye in the non-arteritic form (40–50%).

Optic atrophy (Fig. 14.4)

A pale optic disc represents a loss of nerve fibres at the optic nerve head (Table 14.2). The vision is usually reduced. On examination the usual vascularity of the disc is lost. Comparison of the two eyes is of great help in unilateral cases as the contrast makes identification of pallor much easier. A relative afferent pupillary defect will also be present (see p. 26).

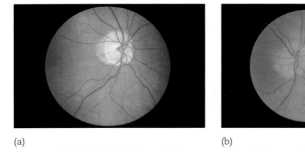

(a)   (b)

Fig. 14.4 (a) A pale optic disc compared to (b) a normal optic disc.

PALE OPTIC DISC

Cause	Distinguishing features
Compression of the optic nerve	History of orbital or chiasmal disease. If sectorial, field loss may give a clue to the location of a compressive lesion.
Ischaemic optic neropathy Retinal artery and vein occlusion	A history of sudden (unilateral) visual loss in the past. The retinal vessels may be attenuated.
Glaucoma (see Chapter 10)	The optic disc is pathologically cupped.
Optic neuritis	There may be a history of previous loss of vision. Symptoms and signs compatible with multiple sclerosis may be present.
Inherited optic nerve disease	Dominant and recessive optic neuropathy are associated with onset of blindness in the first few years of life. Leber's optic neuropathy results from an inheritable mutation of mitochondrial DNA. Onset is typically in early adulthood. It is bilateral. The optic disc appears pale.
Inherited retinal disease	Retinal disease may result in optic disc pallor. It is, for example, a feature of rod-cone dystrophies and retinitis pigmentosa.
Toxic optic neuropathy	Optic neuropathy may follow chemical toxicity for example heavy metals, toluene from glue sniffing and some drugs (i.e. isoniazid used in the treatment of TB). Again information should be sought in the history.
Tobacco-alcohol, nutritional Vitamin amblyopia	Optic neuropathy here (where all three factors are often involved together) is due to a combination of vitamin deficiency (B_{12}) and cyanide toxicity.

Table 14.2 Causes of a pale optic disc.

THE CHIASM

Compressive lesions at the chiasm produce a bitemporal hemianopia as the fibres representing the nasal retina (temporal field) are compressed as they cross in the centre of the chiasm. Patients may present with rather vague visual symptoms, e.g.:

- missing objects in the periphery of the visual field;
- when testing vision with a Snellen chart patients may miss the temporal letters with each eye;
- the bitemporal field loss may cause difficulty in fusing images causing the patient to complain of diplopia although eye movements are normal;
- there may be difficulty with tasks requiring stereopsis such as pouring water into a cup or threading a needle.

The most common lesion is a pituitary tumour and the patient should be asked for symptoms relating to hormonal disturbance (Fig. 14.5). Treatment depends on the type of tumour found, some are amenable to medical therapy but many require surgical excision. A *meningioma* and *craniopharyngioma* may also cause chiasmal compression.

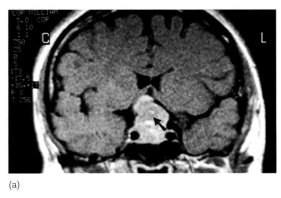

(a)

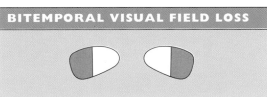

Fig. 14.5 (a) The CT appearance of a pituitary tumour. (b) The bitemporal visual field loss produced.

(b)

OPTIC TRACT, RADIATION AND VISUAL CORTEX (Fig. 14.6)

Lesions (usually either vascular or neoplastic) of the optic tract and radiation produce a *homonymous hemianopic field defect*, that is, loss confined to the right or left-hand side of the field in both eyes. This pattern of field loss results from the crossing of the fibres representing the nasal retina in the chiasm. If the extent of field loss is similar in both eyes a *congruous* defect is said to be present. This usually means that the defect has affected the optic radiation or cerebral cortex. Neoplasia more commonly affects the radiation in the anterior temporal lobe. The commonest cause of disease in the occipital cortex is a cerebrovascular accident. The visual loss is of rapid onset, a slower onset is suggestive of a space occupying lesion.

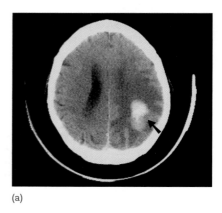

(a)

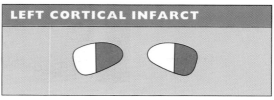

LEFT CORTICAL INFARCT

(b)

Fig. 14.6 (a) A CT scan showing a left cortical infarct. (b) The incomplete congruous right homonymous hemianopia produced by the infarct.

KEY POINTS

- A bitemporal visual field defect suggests a pituitary lesion.
- There are several causes of a swollen optic disc, it is not just a sign of raised intraocular pressure.
- A pale optic disc may result from retinal disease.

Box 14.1 Key points in disease of the optic pathway.

CHAPTER 15

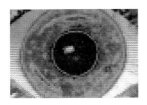

Eye movements

INTRODUCTION

Eye movements may be abnormal because there is:
- an abnormal position of the eyes;
- a reduced range of eye movement;
- an abnormality in the form of eye movement.

ANATOMY AND PHYSIOLOGY (Fig. 15.1)

Each eye can be *abducted* (away from the nose) or *adducted* (towards the nose) or may look up (*elevation*) or down (*depression*). The cardinal positions of gaze for assessing a muscle palsy are: gaze right, left, up, down, and gaze to the right and left in the up and down positions.

Six extraocular muscles control eye movement. The medial and lateral recti bring about horizontal eye movements causing adduction and abduction respectively. The vertical recti elevate and depress the eye in abduction. The superior oblique causes depression in the adducted position and the inferior oblique causes elevation in the adducted position. The vertical muscles all have additional secondary actions (intorsion and extorsion (circular movement of the eye).

Three cranial nerves supply these muscles (see p. 15) whose nuclei are found in the brainstem, together with connections linking them with other nuclei (e.g. vestibular) and with gaze centres (horizontal gaze in the pons and vertical gaze in the midbrain). These coordinate the movements of both eyes.

Higher cortical centres control the speed of the eyes in following a moving target (*pursuit*), and the rapid movements required to take up another position of gaze (*saccades*). These centres also influence the brainstem nuclei.

The linkage of the nuclei ensures that the eyes move together in a coordinated way. For example when looking to the right, the right lateral and left medial rectus are equally stimulated (they are said to be *yoke muscles*). At the same time innervation of the antagonists which move

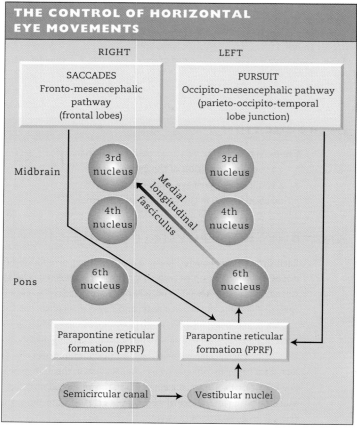

Fig. 15.1 The connections of the nuclei and higher centres controlling horizontal eye movements.

the eyes to the left, (the left lateral rectus and the right medial rectus) is inhibited.

Clinically, eye movement disorders are best described under four headings (which are not mutually exclusive):

1 In a *non-paralytic squint* the movements of both eyes are full (there is no paresis) but only one eye is directed towards the fixated target (Fig. 15.2). The angle of deviation is constant and unrelated to the direction of gaze. This is also termed a *concomitant squint* and is the squint that is seen in childhood.

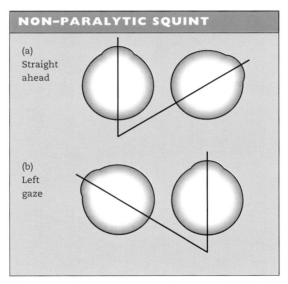

NON–PARALYTIC SQUINT

(a) Straight ahead

(b) Left gaze

Fig. 15.2 The pattern of eye movement seen in a non-paralytic squint: (a) the right eye is divergent in the primary position of gaze (looking straight ahead); (b) when the eyes look to the left the angle of deviation between the *visual axis* (a line passing through the point of fixation and the foveola) of the two eyes is unchanged.

2 In a *paralytic squint* there is underaction of one or more of the eye muscles due to a nerve palsy, extraocular muscle disease or tethering of the globe. The size of the squint is dependent on the direction of gaze and, for a nerve palsy, is greatest in the *field of action* (the direction in which the muscle would normally take the globe) of the affected muscle. This is also termed an *inconcomitant squint*.

3 In gaze palsies there is a disturbance of the supranuclear coordination of eye movements, pursuit and saccadic eye movements may also be

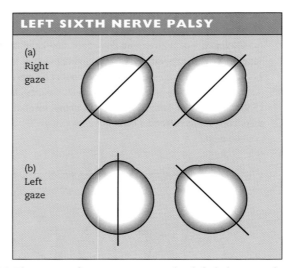

LEFT SIXTH NERVE PALSY

(a)
Right
gaze

(b)
Left
gaze

Fig. 15.3 The pattern of eye movement seen in a left sixth nerve palsy with paralysis of the left lateral rectus. (a) The eyes are looking to the right, the visual axes are aligned, there is no deviation between the visual axes of the two eyes. (b) The eyes look to the left (the field of action of the left lateral rectus). The left lateral rectus is paralyzed and thus the left eye is unable to move past the midline. Now there is a marked angle of deviation between the visual axes of the two eyes.

affected if the cortical pathways to the nuclei controlling eye movements are interrupted (Fig. 15.3).

4 Disorders of the brainstem nuclei or vestibular input may also result in a form of oscillating eye movement termed *nystagmus*.

NON-PARALYTIC SQUINT

Binocular single vision (Fig. 15.4)

In the absence of a squint the eyes are directed towards the same object. Their movements are coordinated so that the retinal images of an object fall on corresponding points of each retina. These images are fused centrally, so that they are interpreted by the brain as a single image. This is termed *binocular single vision*. Because each eye views an object from a different angle, the retinal images do not correspond precisely; the closer the object the greater this disparity. These differences allow a three dimensional percept to be constructed. This is termed *stereopsis*. The development of stereopsis requires that eye movements and visual alignment are coordinated in approximately the first five years of life.

Binocular single vision and stereopsis afford certain advantages to the individual:

- they increase the field of vision;
- they eliminate the blind spot, since the blind spot of one eye falls in the seeing field of the other;
- they provide a binocular acuity which is greater than monocular acuity;
- stereopsis provides depth perception.

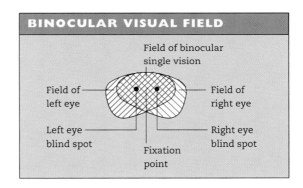

Fig. 15.4 Elimination of the blind spot and increase in the field of vision that binocular single vision affords.

If the visual axes of the two eyes are not aligned, binocular single vision is not possible. This results in:

- *Diplopia*. An object is seen to be in two different places.
- *Visual confusion*. Two separate and different objects appear to be at the same point.

In children, a non-alignment of the visual axes of the two eyes (or squint) results in suppression of the image in the squinting eye. This means that when the vision in the two eyes is tested together only one object is seen. If this is prolonged and constant it causes a reduced visual acuity in the squinting eye (*strabismic amblyopia*) when the vision is tested separately in each eye. Amblyopia will only develop if the squint constantly affects the same eye. Some children alternate the squinting eye. These children will not develop amblyopia, but they do not develop stereopsis either.

Aetiology of non-paralytic squint (Fig. 15.5)

Non-paralytic squint:

1 May develop in an otherwise normal child with normal eyes. The cause of the problem in these patients remains obscure. It is thought to be caused by an abnormality in the central coordination of eye movements.

2 May be associated with ocular disease:

(a) A refractive error which prevents the formation of a clear image on the retina. This is the most common factor. If the refractive error is dissimilar in the two eyes (*anisometropia*) one retinal image will be blurred.

(b) Opacities in the media of the eye blurring or preventing the formation of the retinal image (i.e. corneal opacities or cataract).

(c) Abnormalities of the retina preventing the translation of a correctly formed image into neural impulses.

(d) In a child equally long sighted (hypermetropic) in both eyes a convergent squint may develop because the increased accommodation of the lens (which will correct the hypermetropic error) needed to achieve a clear retinal image for distant objects (and even more for near) will be associated with excessive convergence. Here squint may only occur on attempted convergence, in which case amblyopia does not develop since binocular visual alignment remains normal for some of the time during distant viewing.

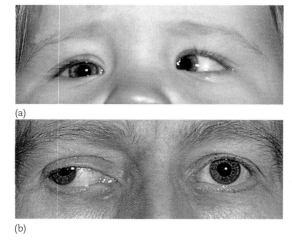

(a)

(b)

Fig. 15.5 The appearance of: (a) a convergent; (b) a divergent squint.

HISTORY

The presence of a squint in a child may be noted by the parents or detected at pre-school or school screening clinics. It may be intermittent or constant. There may be a family history of squint or refractive error. The following should be noted:

- when the squint is present;
- how long a squint has been present for;
- past medical, birth and family history of the child.

EXAMINATION

First the patient is observed for features that may simulate a squint. These include:

- epicanthus (a crescentic fold of skin on the side of the nose that incompletely covers the inner canthus);
- facial asymmetry.

The corneal reflection of a pen torch held 33 cm in front of the subject is a guide to eye position. If the child is squinting the reflection will be central in the fixating eye and deviated in the squinting eye.

A *cover/uncover test* (Fig. 15.6) is next performed to detect a manifest squint (a *tropia*).

- The right eye is completely covered for a few seconds whilst holding a detailed near target (usually a small picture or a toy) in front of the subject as a fixation target. The left eye is closely observed. If it has been maintaining fixation it should not move.
- The cover is removed from the right eye and the left eye covered, this time closely observing the right. If it has been maintaining fixation it should not move. If it has not been maintaining fixation it will move to take up fixation. If it moves *outwards* to take up fixation an *esotropia* or convergent squint is present. If it moves *inwards* to take up fixation an *exotropia* is present.

The test is repeated for a distance object sited at 6 metres and for a far distant object. It will also reveal a vertical squint.

If no abnormal eye movement is seen an *alternate cover test* is performed. This will reveal the presence of a latent squint (a *phoria*), that is one which occurs only in the absence of bifoveal visual stimulation. It is not really an abnormal condition and can be demonstrated in most people who otherwise have normal binocular single vision.

This time the cover is moved rapidly from one eye to the other a couple of times. This dissociates the eyes (there is no longer bifoveal stimulation). The right eye is now occluded and as the occluder is removed any movement in the *right* eye is noted. If the eye is seen to move inwards an *exophoria* (latent divergence) is present and the eye has moved inwards to take up fixation. If the eye is seen to move outwards to take up fixation an *esophoria* (latent convergence) is present. Exactly the same movements would be seen in the left eye if it were covered following dissociation.

In an eye clinic the squint can be further assessed with the synoptophore (see p. 32). This instrument together with special three-

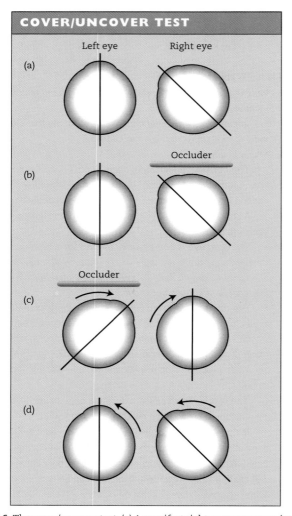

Fig. 15.6 The cover/uncover test. (a) A manifest right convergent squint (right esotropia) is present. (b) The right, squinting eye, is occluded. There is no movement of the left eye which maintains fixation. (c) The left eye is occluded, the squinting right eye moves outwards to take up fixation, the non-squinting eye moves inwards because the movement of the two eyes is linked. (d) The cover is removed from the left eye which moves outwards to take up fixation, the right eye moves inward to resume its squinting position. (If an alternating squint was present (i.e. each eye retained the ability to fixate) the right eye would maintain fixation and the eyes would not move when the cover was removed.

dimensional pictures can also be used to determine whether the eyes are used together and whether stereopsis is present.

Refractive error is measured (following topical administration of atropine or cyclopentolate eye drops to paralyse accommodation and dilate the pupil). The eye is then examined to exclude opacities of the cornea, lens or vitreous and abnormalities of the retina or optic disc.

INVESTIGATING A SQUINT

Examination
• Determination of acuity (see p. 20).
• Detection of any abnormality in eye movement.
• Detection and measurement of squint.
• Measurement of stereopsis.
• Determination of any refractive error.
• Careful examination of the eyes including dilated fundus view.

Box 15.1 Summary of the steps taken in investigating a squinting child.

TREATMENT

A non-paralytic squint with no associated ocular disease is treated as follows:
• Any significant refractive error is first corrected with glasses.
• If amblyopia is present and the vision does not improve with glasses the better seeing eye is patched to try and stimulate the amblyopic eye thereby increasing its visual acuity.
• *Surgical intervention* to realign the eyes may be required for functional reasons (to restore or establish binocular single vision) or for cosmetic reasons (to prevent a child being singled out at school) (Fig. 15.7).

The principle of surgery is to realign the eyes by adjusting the position of the muscles on the globe or by shortening the muscle. Access to the muscles is gained by making a small incision in the conjunctiva.
• Moving the muscle insertion backwards on the globe (*recession*) weakens the muscle.
• Removing a segment of the muscle (*resection*) strengthens the action.

PROGNOSIS

Glasses and patching can significantly improve vision in the squinting eye. Unfortunately realignment, even if performed when the child is very young, is rarely associated with the development of stereopsis in the majority of non-paralytic squints. The operation is important from the cosmetic viewpoint, however, particularly when the child starts school.

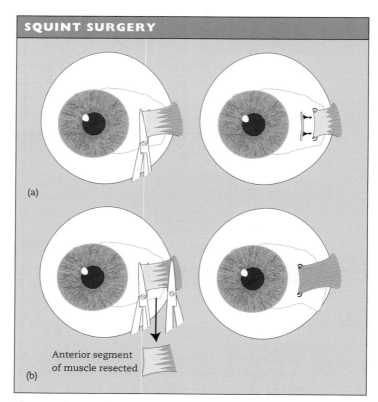

SQUINT SURGERY

(a)

(b)

Anterior segment
of muscle resected

Fig. 15.7 Diagramatic illustration of the principles of squint surgery. (a) Recession. The conjunctiva has been incised to expose the medial rectus muscle. The muscle is then disinserted and moved backwards on the globe. (b) Resection. Following exposure of the muscle the anterior tendon and muscle is resected, thus shortening the muscle, the muscle is then reattached to its original position.

PARALYTIC SQUINT

Isolated nerve palsy (Fig. 15.8)

PATHOGENESIS

Disease of the third, fourth and sixth nerves and their central connections gives rise to a paralytic strabismus. Each nerve may be affected at any point along its course from brainstem nucleus to orbit. Table 15.1 details some causes.

ISOLATED NERVE PALSIES

Orbital disease	(e.g. neoplasia)
Vascular Disease	Diabetes (a 'pupil sparing' third nerve palsy, i.e. there is no mydriasis). Hypertension Aneurysm (most commonly a *painful third nerve palsy* from an aneurysm of the posterior communicating artery. Mydriasis is usually present.) Carotid-cavernous sinus fistula Cavernous sinus thrombosis
Trauma	(Most common cause of fourth and sixth nerve palsy)
Neoplasia	Meningioma Acoustic neuroma Glioma
Raised intracranial pressure	May cause a third or sixth palsy (a false localizing sign)
Inflammation	Sarcoidosis Vasculitic disease (i.e. giant cell arteritis) Infection (particularly herpes zoster) Guillain–Barré syndrome

Table 15.1 The cause of isolated nerve palsies.

HISTORY AND EXAMINATION

The patient complains of diplopia. There may be an abnormal head posture to compensate for the inability of the eye to move in a particular direction. A third nerve palsy results in:

- failure of adduction, elevation and depression of the eye;
- ptosis;
- in some cases, a dilated pupil due to involvement of the autonomic fibres.

A fourth nerve palsy results in defective depression of the eye when attempted in adduction.

It produces the least noticeable eye movement abnormality. Patients may notice vertical double vision with some torsion of the image particularly when going downstairs or reading.

A sixth nerve palsy results in failure of abduction of the eye.

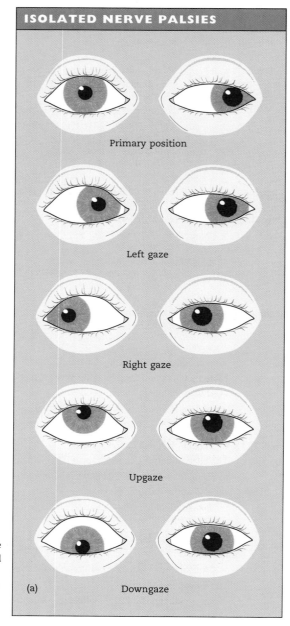

ISOLATED NERVE PALSIES

Primary position

Left gaze

Right gaze

Upgaze

(a)   Downgaze

Fig. 15.8 (a) Left third nerve palsy. Note the dilated pupil and ptosis (not shown) as well as the limitation of eye movement. (*Continued opposite.*)

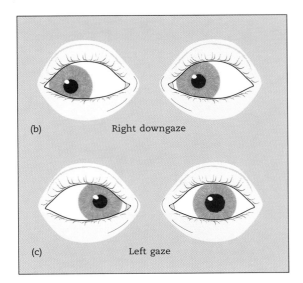

(b) Right downgaze

(c) Left gaze

Fig. 15.8 (*Continued.*)
(b) Left fourth nerve palsy, the defect is maximal when the patient tries to look down when the left eye is adducted. (c) Sixth nerve palsy, the left eye is unable to abduct.

TREATMENT

An isolated nerve palsy is often related to coexistent systemic disease. If a posterior communicating aneurysm is suspected the patient must be sent for neurosurgical review and angiography. The most common cause of a palsy is microvascular disease of the peripheral cranial nerve, itself associated with diabetes or hypertension. Here, nerve function recovers over some months and the symptoms abate.

Orbital disease (see p. 40) and disease in the cavernous sinus may also be the cause of multiple nerve palsies as the third, fourth and sixth nerves become anatomically close together. A CT or MRI scan will show the lesion (e.g. an orbital metastasis).

Diplopia can be helped by fitting prisms to the patients' glasses which realign the retinal images. Alternatively the affected eye can be patched. If eye movements fail to improve spontaneously then surgical intervention may be required. Such intervention will seldom restore normal eye movement but is aimed at restoring an acceptable binocular single vision in the primary positions of gaze (i.e. straight ahead and in downgaze), the commonest positions in which the eyes are used.

DISEASE OF THE EXTRAOCULAR MUSCLES

Dysthyroid eye disease (Fig. 15.9)

PATHOGENESIS

Disorders of the thyroid gland can be associated with an infiltration of the extraocular muscles with lymphocytes and the deposition of glycosamino-glycans. An immunological process is suspected but not fully determined.

SYMPTOMS AND SIGNS

The patient may sometimes complain of:
- A red painful eye (associated with exposure caused by proptosis). If the redness is limited to part of the eye only it may indicate active inflammation in the adjacent muscle.
- Double vision.
- Reduced visual acuity (sometimes associated with optic neuropathy).
  On examination:
- There may be *proptosis* of the eye (the eye protrudes from the orbit, also termed *exophthalmos*).
- The eye may be *chemosed* and injected over the muscle insertions.
- The upper lid may be *retracted* so that sclera is visible (thought to be due in part to increased sympathetic activity stimulating the sympathetically innervated smooth muscle of levator). This results in a characteristic stare.
- The upper lid may lag behind the movement of the globe on downgaze (*lid lag*).
- There may be restricted eye movements or squint, (also termed restrictive thyroid myopathy, exophthalmic ophthalmoplegia, dysthyroid eye disease or Graves' disease).

The inferior rectus is the most commonly affected muscle. Its movement becomes restricted and there is mechanical limitation of the eye in upgaze. Involvement of the medial rectus causes mechanical limitation of abduction thereby mimicking a sixth nerve palsy. A CT or MRI scan shows enlargement of the muscles.

Dysthyroid eye disease is associated with two serious acute complications:

I   Excessive exposure of the conjunctiva and cornea with the formation of chemosis (oedematous swelling of the conjunctiva), and corneal ulcers due to proptosis and failure of the lids to protect the cornea. The condition may lead to corneal perforation.

2   Compressive optic neuropathy due to compression and ischaemia of the optic nerve by the thickened muscles. This leads to field loss and may cause blindness.

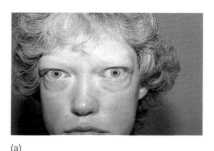

(a)

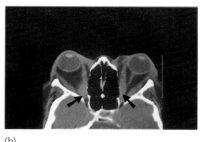

(b)

Fig. 15.9 (a) The clinical appearance of dysthyroid eye disease; (b) a CT scan demonstrating muscle thickening.

TREATMENT

Corneal exposure and optic nerve compression require urgent treatment with systemic steroids, radiotherapy or surgical orbital decompression.

In the long term, treatment may be needed for the eye movement problems and to improve the cosmetic appearance of the eyes. A period may elapse while the eye movements stabilize, during which time prisms can be added to manage the diplopia. Once stabilized, if the patient remains symptomatic, surgery on the extraocular muscles can be performed to increase the field of binocular single vision. If desired cosmetic surgery to lower the lids can also be performed following the squint surgery.

Myasthenia gravis

PATHOGENESIS

Myasthenia gravis is caused by the development of antibodies to the acetylcholine receptors of striated muscle. It affects females more than males and although commonest in the 15–50 age group may affect young children and older adults. Some 40% of patients may show involvement of the extraocular muscles only.

SYMPTOMS AND SIGNS

The extraocular muscles fatigue resulting in a variable diplopia. A variable ptosis may also be present. This can be demonstrated by asking the patient to look up and down a number of times to fatigue the muscle. There may be evidence of systemic muscle weakness.

TREATMENT

The diagnosis can be confirmed by electromyography or by determining whether an injection of neostigmine or edrophonium temporarily restores normal muscle movement (this test must be performed under close medical supervision with resuscitation equipment and atropine to hand because of the possibility of cholinergic side effects such as bradycardia and bronchospasm.).

Patients are treated, in conjunction with a neurologist, with neostigmine or pyridostigmine. Systemic steroids and surgical removal of the thymus also have a role in treatment.

Ocular myositis

This is an inflammation of the extraocular muscles associated with pain and diplopia, leading to a restriction in the movement of the involved muscle (similar to that seen in dysthyroid eye disease). It is not usually associated with systemic disease but thyroid abnormalities should be excluded. The conjunctiva over the involved muscle is inflamed. CT or MRI scanning shows a thickening of the muscle. If symptoms are troublesome it responds to a short course of steroids.

Ocular myopathy

Ocular myopathy (progressive external ophthalmoplegia) is a rare condition where the movement of the eyes is slowly and symmetrically reduced. There is an associated ptosis. Ultimately, eye movement may be lost completely.

Brown's syndrome

The action of the superior oblique muscle may be congenitally restricted which reduces elevation of the eye when it is adducted (Brown's syndrome). The exact cause remains unknown although it may involve an abnormality of the tendon as it passes through the trochlear. The condition may also result from trauma to the orbit.

Duane's syndrome

This is a 'congenital miswiring' of the medial and lateral rectus muscles, (cases of an absent sixth nerve and nucleus are also reported). There is neuromuscular activity in the lateral rectus during adduction and reduced lateral rectus activity in abduction. This results in limited abduction and apparent narrowing of the palpebral aperture on adduction with retraction of the eye into the globe (due to contraction of both medial and laternal rectus muscles). The condition may be unilateral or, more rarely, bilateral. Children do not usually develop amblyopia and surgical intervention is often not required.

GAZE PALSIES

Disordered eye movement results from damage to the pathways connecting the cranial nerve nuclei and the higher centres. The abnormality in eye movements depends on the point at which the pathway is disrupted. Both the extent and form of eye movement may be affected. Some of the more common are briefly described below. The ophthalmologist usually investigates and manages these patients with the help of a neurologist.

Lesions of the parapontine reticular formation (PPRF)

PATHOGENESIS

The PPRF controls the horizontal movements of the eyes. Lesions affecting the PPRF are usually associated with other brainstem disease. It may be seen in patients with:

- vascular disease;
- tumours.

SYMPTOMS AND SIGNS

There is:

- a failure of horizontal movements of both eyes to the side of the lesion (a *horizontal gaze palsy*);
- deviation of the eyes to the contralateral side in acute cases.

Internuclear ophthalmoplegia (Fig. 15.10)

PATHOGENESIS

It is caused by a lesion of the medial longitudinal fasiculus (MLF). The MLF joins the sixth nerve nucleus to the third nerve nucleus on the opposite side.

It may become damaged in:

- demyelination (usually bilateral);
- vascular disease (unilateral).

SYMPTOMS AND SIGNS

The patient complains of horizontal diplopia.
There is a:
- reduction of adduction on the same side as the lesion.
- nystagmus of the contralateral, abducting eye.

MANAGEMENT

Spontaneous recovery is usual. An MRI scan may be helpful diagnostically both to locate the causal brainstem lesion and, in demyelination, to determine whether other plaques are present.

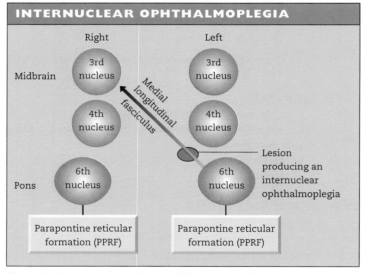

Fig. 15.10 Diagram showing the site of the lesion producing an internuclear ophthalmoplegia.

Parinaud's syndrome (dorsal midbrain syndrome)

PATHOGENESIS

In Parinaud's syndrome a lesion exists in the dorsal midbrain involving the centre for vertical gaze. It may be seen in patients with:

- demyelination;
- space occupying lesions such as a pinealoma which press on the tectum;
- infarction of the dorsal midbrain;
- an enlarged third ventricle.

SYMPTOMS AND SIGNS

The disorder causes:
- deficient elevation of both eyes;
- convergence of the eyes and retraction into the orbit associated with nystagmus on attempted elevation;
- light-near dissociation of the pupil (the pupil constricts on accommodation but reacts poorly to a light stimulus).

ABNORMAL OSCILLATIONS OF THE EYES

Nystagmus

This refers to repeated involuntary to and fro or up and down movements of the eyes. Similar movements may occur normally when following a moving object (e.g. looking out of a train window) (*optokinetic nystagmus*) or following stimulation of the vestibular system. When examined closely they may be seen to have a slow phase in one direction and a fast phase in the other (*jerk nystagmus*). The nystagmus is described as beating to the side of the fast component. In some cases the speed of eye movement may be roughly the same in either direction (*pendular nystagmus*). Jerk nystagmus may also be seen at the extreme position of gaze (*end gaze nystagmus*).

ACQUIRED NYSTAGMUS

Pathologically, jerk nystagmus may be seen:
- In cerebellar disease, when it is worse when gaze is directed towards the side of the lesion. The fast movement is directed towards the side of the lesion.
- With some drugs (such as barbiturates).
- In damage to the labyrinth and its central connections when a fine jerk nystagmus results. The fast phase of the movement is away from the lesion and it is usually present only acutely.

An upbeat nystagmus (fast phase upwards) is commonly associated with brainstem disease. It may also be seen in toxic states, e.g. in excess alcohol intake.

A downbeat nystagmus may be seen in patients with a posterior fossa lesion near the cervicomedullary junction (e.g. a Chiari malformation where cerebellar tissue passes through the foramen magnum). It may also be seen in patients with demyelination and again may be present in toxic states.

Patients with nerve palsies or weakness of the extraocular muscles may develop nystagmus when looking in the direction of the affected muscle (*gaze-evoked nystagmus*). The fast phase of the movement is in the field of action of the weak muscle.

Patients with acquired nystagmus complain that the visual environment is in continual movement (*oscillopsia*).

CONGENITAL NYSTAGMUS

Nystagmus can be congenital in origin.

• Sensory congenital nystagmus. Here the movements may be at similar speeds in both directions (*pendular nystagmus*) or of the jerk variety. It is associated with poor vision (e.g. congenital cataract, albinism).

• Motor congenital nystagmus is a jerk nystagmus developing at birth in children with no visual defect.

The continuous movement of the eye reduces visual acuity but does not cause oscillopsia in congenital nystagmus. The exact degree of disability depends on:

• the speed of the nystagmus;

• whether there are short periods of rest between the nystagmoid movements when objects can be focused on the fovea;

• whether the nystagmus is reduced by accommodation as is often the case.

Some subjects find a position of the eyes which reduces the nystagmus to a minimum (the null position), thus maximising visual acuity.

KEY POINTS

• In analysing eye movement problems try to determine whether there is a reduction in the range of eye movements, an abnormal position of the eyes, an abnormality in the form of eye movement or a combination of these disorders.

• An abnormality in the range of eye movements may reflect muscular, orbital, infranuclear or supranuclear disease.

• In a child with a squint it is important to exclude intraocular pathology.

• An intracranial aneurysm may present as a painful third nerve palsy involving the pupil.

Box 15.2 Key points in eye movement disorders.

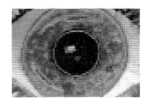

Trauma

INTRODUCTION

Although the eye is well protected in the orbit it may be subject to injuries from which no part is immune (Fig. 16.1). Forms of injury include:

• Foreign bodies becoming lodged under the upper lid or on the surface of the eye, specially the cornea.

• Blunt trauma from objects small enough not to impact on the orbital rim (shuttlecocks, squashballs, champagne corks and knuckles are some of the offenders). The sudden alteration of pressure, and distortion of the eye may cause severe damage.

• Penetrating trauma where ocular structures are damaged by a foreign body which passes through the ocular coat and may also be retained in the eye. With the introduction of the seat belt laws the incidence of penetrating injury following road traffic accidents has declined.

• Chemical and radiation injury where the resultant reaction of the ocular tissues causes the damage.

HISTORY, SYMPTOMS AND SIGNS

A careful history is essential:

• Use of a hammer and chisel can release a flake of metal which will penetrate the globe, leaving only a tell-tale subconjunctival haemorrhage to indicate penetration of the sclera and suggest a retained foreign body.

• A wire under tension, or a rose thorn, may penetrate the cornea briefly, sometimes creating only a barely visible track.

• A blunt injury to the eye may also result in damage to the orbit (*blow-out fracture*).

• It is vitally important to determine the nature of any chemical that may have been in contact with the eye. Strong alkalis penetrate the anterior tissues of the eye and may rapidly cause irreversible damage.

The patient's symptoms will relate to the degree and type of trauma suffered. Pain, lacrimation and blurring of vision are common features of trauma but mild symptoms may disguise a potentially blinding intraocular foreign body. As in all history taking it is essential to enquire about previous ocular and medical history.

EXAMINATION

Without a slit lamp

The examination will depend on the type of injury. In all cases it is impor-

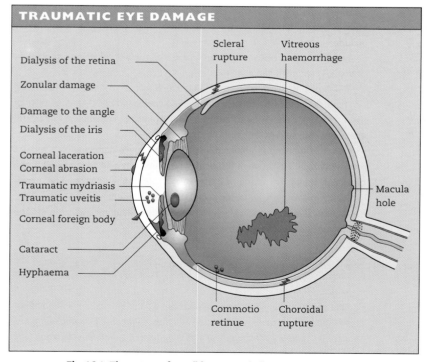

TRAUMATIC EYE DAMAGE

Dialysis of the retina

Zonular damage

Damage to the angle

Dialysis of the iris

Corneal laceration
Corneal abrasion

Traumatic mydriasis
Traumatic uveitis

Corneal foreign body

Cataract

Hyphaema

Scleral rupture

Vitreous haemorrhage

Macula hole

Commotio retinue

Choroidal rupture

Fig. 16.1 The extent of possible traumatic damage to the eye.

tant that visual acuity is recorded in the injured and *uninjured* eye. Where a penetrating injury is suspected and pressure to the globe must be avoided, it may only be possible to measure an approximate vision in the injured eye. The skin around the orbit and eyelids should be carefully examined for a penetrating wound.

ORBITAL INJURY

Damage to the orbit itself (a *blow-out fracture*; Fig. 16.2) is suspected if the following signs are present:

• Emphysema (air in the skin which crackles when pressed) derived from a fractured sinus.

• Areas of paraesthesia suggesting that the infraorbital or supra-orbital nerves have been damaged. The infraorbital nerve is commonly injured in orbital blow-out injury involving the floor of the orbit.

• Limitation of eye movements, particularly on upgaze and downgaze due to tethering of the inferior rectus muscle by connective tissue septa

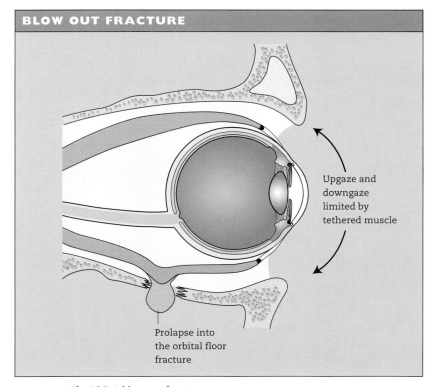

BLOW OUT FRACTURE

Upgaze and downgaze limited by tethered muscle

Prolapse into the orbital floor fracture

Fig. 16.2 A blow-out fracture.

caught on the fractured bone (the inferior orbital floor is the most commonly fractured).

• Subsequently the eye may become recessed into the orbit (*enophthalmos*).

• If the lid margin is cut at the medial canthus it is important to determine if either of the lacrimal canaliculi are involved.

Further examination of a traumatized eye will require the instillation of a local anaesthetic to facilitate lid opening (Lignocaine, Amethocaine). If a penetrating eye injury is suspected it is important that no pressure is applied to the globe.

PENETRATING EYE INJURY

• History of high velocity object hitting the eye
• Dark tissue in the cornea or sclera (iris plugging of wound)
• Distortion of the pupil
• Unusually deep anterior chamber
• Cataract
• Vitreous haemorrhage

Box 16.1 Symptoms and signs of a penetrating eye injury.

THE CONJUNCTIVA AND SCLERA

These must be examined for the presence of any lacerations. If the history is appropriate a subconjunctival haemorrhage should be considered to be the potential site of a scleral perforation (Fig. 16.3).

The fundus should be examined with full mydriasis. If a chemical injury has occurred the conjunctiva may appear white and ischaemic (Fig. 16.4). If such changes are extensive, involving the greater part of the limbal circumference, corneal healing is likely to be grossly impaired and there will

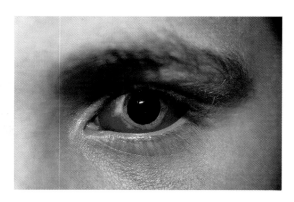

Fig. 16.3 A subconjunctival haemorrhage.

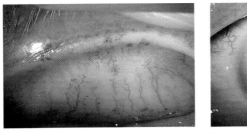
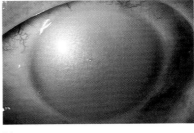

(a)   (b)

Fig. 16.4 (a) Following an alkali burn the upper tarsal conjunctiva has become ischaemic the lid is everted; (b) the cornea following an alkali burn.

be additional complications such as uveitis, secondary glaucoma and cataract.

THE CORNEA

This is examined for loss of the epithelial layer (abrasion) for lacerations and for foreign bodies (Fig. 16.5). The instillation of fluorescein will identify the extent of an abrasion and, if concentrated, will identify a leak of aqueous through a penetrating wound (see p. 28). If the globe appears intact and a subtarsal foreign body is suspected (signalled by fine, vertical, linear corneal abrasions) the upper lid must be everted (see pp. 28–29). This exposes the underside of the lid and allows any foreign body to be identified and removed.

Electromagnetic radiation may injure the conjunctiva and the cornea. Unprotected exposure to ultraviolet light from an arc-lamp (*arc eye*), sunlamp or reflected from snow, is the commonest cause of this severely painful condition. Typically, ocular pain occurs acutely, 6 hours after exposure to the radiation and the cornea shows diffuse epithelial oedema and punctate damage which resolves within 24–48 hours.

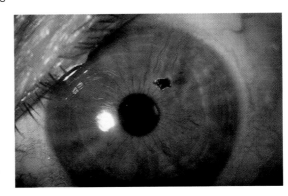

Fig. 16.5 A corneal foreign body. (With permission from Sue Ford, Western Eye Hospital)

THE ANTERIOR CHAMBER

Blunt trauma may cause haemorrhage into the anterior chamber where it collects with a fluid level (*hyphaema*). This is caused by rupture of the root of the iris blood vessels or the iris may be torn away from its insertion into the ciliary body (*iris dialysis*) to produce a D-shaped pupil. Hyphaema may also be seen with a penetrating eye injury, and the shape of the pupil may be distorted if the peripheral iris has plugged a penetrating wound (Fig. 16.6). The pupil may also be dilated as a result of blunt trauma (*traumatic mydriasis*).

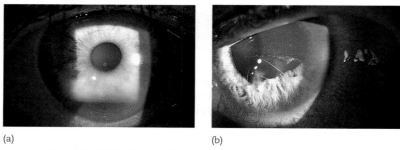

(a)   (b)

Fig. 16.6 (a) A hyphaema; (b) penetrating eye injury (note the eyelashes in the anterior chamber and the distorted iris).

THE LENS

Dislocation of the lens following blunt trauma may be suggested by a fluttering of the iris diaphragm on eye movement (*iridonesis*). Lens clarity should be assessed with the slit lamp and against the red reflex after pupil dilation. Cataracts develop abruptly with direct penetrating trauma (Fig. 16.7). Blunt trauma also causes a posterior subcapsular cataract within hours of injury, which may be transient.

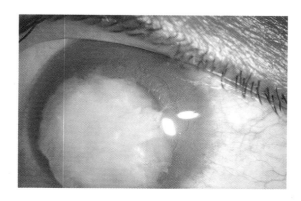

Fig. 16.7 The lens in this patient has become disrupted and cataractous following penetrating trauma.

THE FUNDUS

The fundus should be inspected with a direct ophthalmoscope after full mydriasis. If no neurological complications accompany the injury and an ocular penetration is not suspected, the pupil can be dilated. If no details are visible this suggests a vitreous haemorrhage. Areas of retinal haemorrhage and whiteness (oedema) may be seen (*commotio retinae*). A *retinal dialysis* (a separation of the peripheral retina from its junction with the pars plana of the ciliary body) and a macular hole (see p. 115) may also result from blunt trauma. The choroid may also become torn, acutely this may cause sub-retinal haemorrhage which is followed by the development of sub-retinal scarring. Peripheral retinal changes can only be excluded with indirect ophthalmoscopy or slit lamp microscopy.

With a slit lamp

The slit lamp will allow a more detailed examination to be performed, which may reveal:

• A shallow anterior chamber compared to the fellow eye suggesting anterior penetrating injury.

• A microscopic hyphaema where the red cells are present in the anterior chamber but have not settled to form a hyphaema.

• The presence of white cells in the anterior chamber (*traumatic uveitis*).

• *Recession* of the iridocorneal angle seen with a gonioscopic contact lens (the insertion of ciliary muscle into scleral spur moves posteriorly).

• Raised intraocular pressure measured by applanation tonometry. This may accompany a hyphaema or lens dislocation.

TREATMENT

Lacerations to the skin and lids

These require careful suturing particularly if the lid margin is involved. If one of the lacrimal canaliculi is damaged an attempt can be made to repair it but if repair is unsuccessful usually the remaining tear duct is capable of draining all the tears. If both canaliculi are involved, an attempt at repair should always be made.

Corneal abrasions

These normally heal rapidly and should be treated with antibiotic ointment and an eye pad. Dilatation of the pupil with Cyclopentolate 1% can help to relieve the pain caused by spasm of the ciliary muscle.

Following such injury, usually with flexible objects such as fingernails, twigs or the edge of a newspaper a minority of patients may be troubled by recurrent episodes of pain particularly in the early hours of the morning or on waking. This condition is termed *recurrent corneal erosion* and is due to a defective adhesion of the resurfacing epithelium to Bowman's layer at the site of injury. Symptoms may be temporarily relieved by using a lubricating ointment at night, but more permanent results can be achieved by applying a series of fine *micropunctures* to the affected zone and inducing a scar.

Radiation injury to the cornea responds quickly to the same treatment as an abrasion.

Corneal foreign bodies (Fig. 16.8)

Corneal foreign bodies should be removed with a needle under topical anaesthesia, a rust ring may remain and can be removed with a small burr. Subtarsal objects can often be swept away with a cotton wool bud from the everted lid. The patient is then treated as for an abrasion. If there is any suggestion that a foreign body may have penetrated the globe the eye must be carefully examined with dilation of the pupil to allow a good view of the lens and retina. An X-ray with the eyes looking up and then the eyes looking down or a CT scan may also be indicated if an intraocular foreign body is suspected. Microsurgical techniques can be used to remove foreign bodies from the eye under direct visualization.

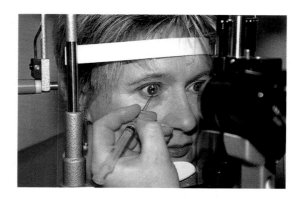

Fig. 16.8 Removal of a superficial ocular foreign body at the slit lamp.

Corneal and scleral penetrating trauma

Once identified no further examination of the globe should be performed but a shield should be gently placed over the eye and the patient referred for urgent ophthalmic treatment. These serious injuries often with grave implications for sight require careful microsurgical suturing to restore the integrity of the globe. Once the eye has settled from this primary repair additional operations are often required to:

• remove a cataract;
• remove a foreign body;
• repair a detached retina or remove the vitreous gel to prevent this happening.

Occasionally, in the longer term, the fellow eye may develop uveitis as a result of an immune response to the release of antigen from the eye (sympathetic ophthalmitis) (see p. 97).

Uveitis

This reponds to the usual treatment with steroids and dilating drops. It may be accompanied by elevated intraocular pressure requiring additional medical treatment.

Hyphaema

This usually settles with rest but a rebleed may occur in the first 5–6 days after injury. Children usually require admission to hospital for a few days while adults can be treated at home provided they can rest and no complications develop. Steroid eye drops are given for a short time together with dilatation of the pupil. The commonest complication is a raised ocular pressure, particularly if there is a secondary bleed, which tends to be more severe than the first. It is for this reason that rest is important. Raised pressure usually responds to medical treatment but occasionally surgical intervention is required. When the hyphaema has settled it is important that the eye is carefully checked for other complications of blunt trauma.

Retinal damage

Commotio retinae. The affected zone opacifies and obscures the underlying choroidal detail. It usually resolves but requires careful observation since retinal holes may develop in affected areas and may lead to subsequent retinal detachment.

Retinal dialysis requires surgical intervention to repair any detached retina.

A vitreous haemorrhage may absorb over several weeks, or may require removal by vitrectomy. An ultrasound scan is useful in detecting associated retinal detachments.

Chemical injury

The most important part of the treatment is to irrigate the eye immediately with copious quantities of clean water. It is also important to irrigate under the upper and lower lid to remove solid particles, e.g. lime. The nature of the chemical can then be ascertained by history and measuring tear pH with litmus paper. Administration of steroid and dilating drops may be required. Vitamin C given both orally and topically may improve healing and topical anticollagenases may be needed.

Orbital blow-out fracture

If a blow-out fracture is suspected, a CT scan will delineate the bony and soft tissue injury. If this is not possible then plain orbital X-rays are performed. Treatment may be delayed until the periorbital swelling has settled. At this later stage the degree of enophthalmos and the limitation of eye movement can be measured. If the enophthalmos is cosmetically unacceptable or eye movements significantly limited then surgical repair of the orbital fracture is indicated. Although some surgeons advocate an early intervention to obtain the best results many patients will require no surgery at all.

PROGNOSIS

The eye heals well following minor trauma and there are rarely long term sequelae save for the recurrent erosion syndrome. Penetrating ocular trauma, however, is often associated with severe visual damage and may require extensive surgery. Long-term retention of iron foreign bodies may destroy retinal function by the generation of free radicals. Similarly, chemical injuries to the eyes can result in severe long-term visual impairment and ocular discomfort. Blunt trauma can cause untreatable visual loss if a retinal hole develops at the fovea. Vision will also be impaired if the choroid at the macula is damaged. In the longer term secondary glaucoma can develop in an eye several years after the initial insult if the trabecular meshwork has been damaged. Severe orbital trauma may also cause both cosmetic and oculomotor problems.

KEY POINTS

- Take an accurate history.
- Foreign bodies can often be found under the upper lid.
- Persistant pain in an intact eye suggests a subtarsal foreign body.
- Irrigate chemical injuries immediately with clean water.
- Suspect a perforating eye injury if the pupil is not round, a cataract has developed rapidly or a vitreous haemorrhage is present.

Box 16.2 Key points in ocular trauma.

CHAPTER 17

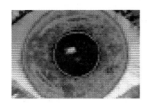

Services for the visually handicapped

INTRODUCTION

Blindness has not been satisfactorily defined. Legally it is said to be, 'so blind as to be unable to perform any work for which sight is essential.' This definition is none too helpful and each case must be assessed on its individual merits. The effects of reduced vision are influenced by:

- The speed and age at which it occurred (sudden visual loss is harder to adjust to than a gradual loss; younger people may be able to adapt better to poor vision than older people.
- Whether central or peripheral vision is affected.
- The type of field defect that is present. Homonymous hemianopia may present special difficulties in reading and navigation.
- The existence of other disabilities (e.g. deafness).

Help and advice is available in the UK both from local government (social services) and voluntary organizations such as the Royal National Institute for the Blind (RNIB). There are also numerous local groups that offer support. Help is aimed at enabling the visually impaired person to lead an independent life.

BLIND REGISTRATION

In the UK, patients with poor vision that meet certain requirements can be registered as either partially sighted or blind, depending on the level of visual deficit. Blind registration does not necessarily mean that the person can see nothing at all. This helps to coordinate the services available for the patient. Not all patients wish to be registered, however, because of an assumed stigma and it is important to discuss the subject fully with the patient. Despite the benefits that may follow registration, some patients regard it as an end to a fight against failing sight rather than a new beginning, managing the problem with all available help. It is important not to dismiss the wishes of these patients in trying to maximize their ability to manage their reduced vision. Registration is performed by an ophthalmologist. The benefits of registration, some only available to patients registered blind, include:

- Financial help (e.g. increased tax allowances, additional income support, severe disablement allowance).
- Help from the social services (e.g. specialist assessment, adaptation of living accommodation).
- Exemption from directory enquiry fees.
- Public transport travel concessions.
- Help with access to work.

Patients with impaired sight whether registered or not may also benefit from the 'talking book and newspaper' schemes which provide extensive recorded material on tape.

SERVICES FOR CHILDREN WITH IMPAIRED SIGHT

Children with impaired sight may require additional help with education or be educated in special schools for the visually handicapped. The local education authority has to make a *statement* of the educational needs of the child. Special visual aids including voice-activated computers and closed-circuit television may help.

In addition children may be eligible for the disability living allowance which may enable parents to claim additional benefits.

ADDITIONAL HELP

As well as low vision aids (see p. 39), various devices are also available ranging from telephones with large number buttons, guides to help a patient place their signature on a cheque, devices that indicate when a cup is filled. Additionally, for some patients, training in the use of a cane or guide dog may aid mobility. Some patients may also benefit from learning Braille.

KEY POINTS

- Ensure that the patient is helped to maximise residual vision.
- Ensure that the patient is aware of support services and if appropriate has been registered partially sighted or blind.
- Ensure that appropriate steps are taken for the education of a poorly sighted child.

Box 17.1 Key points in services for the poorly sighted.

Index

Page numbers in *italics* refer to figures, tables or boxes.